Access your Clinics anywhere you go with our new App!

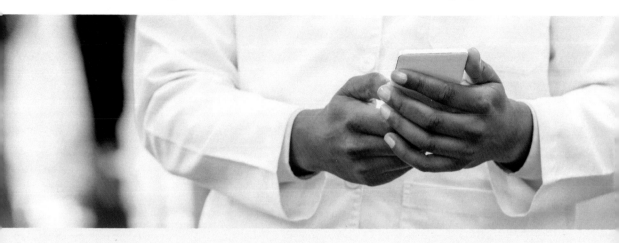

The new and improved Clinics Review Articles mobile app offers subscribers rapid access to recently published content from all Clinics Review Articles titles.

KEY FEATURES OF THE CLINICS APP:

- **Download full issues** while reading – no need to wait!

- **Access articles quickly and conveniently** with new, improved layouts and navigation.

- **Interact with figures, tables, videos**, and other supplementary content.

- **Personalize your experience** by creating reading lists and adding your own notes to articles.

- **Share your favorite articles** on social media and email useful content to colleagues.

DOWNLOAD THE CLINICS APP TODAY!

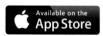 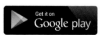

Clinics Review Articles

Prevention, Screening, and Treatments for Obstructive Sleep Apnea: Beyond Positive Airway Pressure (PAP)

Editor

SONG TAR TOH

SLEEP MEDICINE CLINICS

www.sleep.theclinics.com

Consulting Editor
TEOFILO LEE-CHIONG Jr

March 2019 • Volume 14 • Number 1

ELSEVIER

1600 John F. Kennedy Boulevard • Suite 1800 • Philadelphia, Pennsylvania, 19103-2899

http://www.theclinics.com

SLEEP MEDICINE CLINICS Volume 14, Number 1
March 2019, ISSN 1556-407X, ISBN-13: 978-0-323-65529-3

Editor: Colleen Dietzler
Developmental Editor: Donald Mumford

Sleep Medicine Clinics (ISSN 1556-407X) is published quarterly by Elsevier Inc., 360 Park Avenue South, New York, NY 10010-1710. Months of issue are March, June, September and December. Business and Editorial Offices: 1600 John F. Kennedy Blvd., Ste. 1800, Philadelphia, PA 19103-2899. Customer Service Office: 3251 Riverport Lane, Maryland Heights, MO 63043. Periodicals postage paid at New York, NY and additional mailing offices. Subscription prices are $212.00 per year (US individuals), $100.00 (US students), $486.00 (US institutions), $264.00 (Canadian individuals), $252.00 (international individuals) $135.00 (Canadian and international students), $551.00 (Canadian institutions) and $551.00 (International institutions). Foreign air speed delivery is included in all *Clinics* subscription prices. All prices are subject to change without notice. **POSTMASTER:** Send change of address to *Sleep Medicine Clinics*, Elsevier Health Sciences Division, Subscription Customer Service, 3251 Riverport Lane, Maryland Heights, MO 63043. Customer Service: **Tel: 1-800-654-2452 (U.S. and Canada); 314-447-8871 (outside U.S. and Canada). Fax: 314-447-8029. E-mail: journalscustomerservice-usa@elsevier.com (for print support); journalsonlinesupport-usa@elsevier.com (for online support)**.

Reprints. For copies of 100 or more of articles in this publication, please contact the Commercial Reprints Department, Elsevier Inc., 360 Park Avenue South, New York, NY 10010-1710. Tel.: 212-633-3874; Fax: 212-633-3820; E-mail: reprints@elsevier.com.

Sleep Medicine Clinics is covered in *MEDLINE/PubMed (Index Medicus)*.

Printed in the United States of America.

SLEEP MEDICINE CLINICS

SERIES OF RELATED INTEREST

Clinics in Chest Medicine
Available at: https://www.chestmed.theclinics.com/

THE CLINICS ARE AVAILABLE ONLINE!
Access your subscription at:
www.theclinics.com

Contributors

CONSULTING EDITOR

TEOFILO LEE-CHIONG Jr, MD
Professor of Medicine, National Jewish Health,
University of Colorado Denver, Denver,
Colorado, USA; Chief Medical Liaison, Philips
Respironics, Pennsylvania, USA

EDITOR

**SONG TAR TOH, MBBS, MRCSEd, MMED
(ORL), MMED (Sleep Med), FAMS (ORL)**
Senior Consultant, Department of
Otolaryngology, Singapore General Hospital,
Head, Singhealth Duke-NUS Sleep Centre,
Adjunct Associate Professor, National
University of Singapore, Yong Loo Lin School
of Medicine & Duke-NUS Medical School,
Singapore, Singapore

AUTHORS

VICTOR ABDULLAH, MD, PhD
Professor, Department of Otorhinolaryngology,
Head and Neck Surgery (ENT), Chinese
University of Hong Kong, United Christian
Hospital, Hong Kong, China

VIKAS AGRAWAL, MBBS, MS (ENT)
Consultant ENT Surgeon, Head of the
Department of ENT, Specialty ENT Hospital,
Mumbai, Maharashtra, India

MICHAEL AWAD, MD, FRCSC
Fellow, Division of Sleep Surgery,
Department of Otolaryngology, Stanford
University School of Medicine, Stanford,
California, USA

ROBSON CAPASSO, MD
Associate Professor, Co-director of Sleep
Surgery Fellowship, Division of Sleep Surgery,
Department of Otolaryngology, Stanford
University School of Medicine, Stanford,
California, USA

CLEMENT CHENG-HUI LIN, MD, MS
Plastic and Reconstructive Surgeon,
Assistant Professor, Department of Plastic
and Reconstructive Surgery, Craniofacial
Center, Craniofacial Research Center,
Chang Gung Memorial Hospital, College
of Medicine, Chang Gung University,
Taoyuan, Taiwan

KHAI BENG CHONG, MBBS
Department of Otorhinolaryngology,
Tan Tock Seng Hospital, Singapore,
Singapore

LI-CHUAN CHUANG, DDS, MS
Department of Pediatric Dentistry,
Chang Gung Memorial Hospital,
Graduate Institute of Craniofacial and
Dental Science, College of Medicine,
Chang Gung University, Taoyuan,
Taiwan

ANDREA DE VITO, MD, PhD
Consultant, Head and Neck Department, ENT and Oral Surgery Unit, G.B. Morgagni - L. Pierantoni Hospital, AUSL of Romagna, Forlì, Italy

MICHAEL FRIEDMAN, MD, FACS
Professor and Director, Division of Sleep Surgery, Department of Otolaryngology–Head and Neck Surgery, Rush University Medical Center, Professor and Chairman, Department of Otolaryngology, Advanced Center for Specialty Care, Advocate Illinois Masonic Medical Center, Chicago, Illinois, USA

YAU HONG GOH, MD, PhD
Consultant, Department of Otorhinolaryngology–Head and Neck Surgery, Mount Elizabeth Medical Centre, Singapore, Singapore

CHRISTIAN GUILLEMINAULT, DM, MD, DBiol
Division of Sleep Medicine, Stanford University, Redwood City, California, USA

CLEMENS HEISER, MD
Associate Professor, Department of Otorhinolaryngology, Head and Neck Surgery, Klinikum Rechts der Isar, Technische Universitat Munchen, Munich, Germany

BENEDIKT HOFAUER, MD
Department of Otorhinolaryngology, Head and Neck Surgery, Klinikum Rechts der Isar, Technische Universitat Munchen, Munich, Germany

SHIH-CHIEH HSU, MD
Department of Psychiatry and Sleep Center, Chang Gung Memorial Hospital, College of Medicine, Taoyuan, Taiwan

YU-SHU HUANG, MD, PhD
Division of Child Psychiatry and Pediatric Sleep Laboratory, Department of Psychiatry, Chang Gung Memorial Hospital, College of Medicine, Taoyuan, Taiwan

SUNG WAN KIM, MD, PhD
Professor, Department of Otorhinolaryngology–Head and Neck Surgery, Kyung Hee University Hospital, Seoul, Korea

HUNG TUAN LAU, MBBS, MRCS, MMED (ORL)
Otolaryngologist from Singapore, Department of Plastic and Reconstructive Surgery, Clinical Fellow, Craniofacial Center, Chang Gung Memorial Hospital, Taoyuan, Taiwan; Department of Otolaryngology (ENT)–Head and Neck Surgery, Khoo Teck Puat Hospital, Singapore, Singapore

PHONG CHING LEE, MBCHB, FRCP (EDIN)
Consultant, Department of Endocrinology, Singapore General Hospital, Singapore, Singapore

TAN KAH LEONG ALVIN, MBChB, MRCS
Adjunct Assistant Professor, Principal Staff Registrar, Department of Otorhinolaryngology, Head and Neck Surgery, Changi General Hospital, Singapore, Singapore

HSUEH-YU LI, MD, FACS
Professor, Department of Otolaryngology, Chang Gung Memorial Hospital, Professor, School of Medicine, Chang Gung University, President, Taiwan Society of Sleep Medicine, President, Taiwan Voice Society, Executive Council, Taiwan Society of Otolaryngology Head and Neck Surgery, Taoyuan, Taiwan

CHIN HONG LIM, MB, BH, BAO, FRCA
Consultant, Department of Upper Gastrointestinal and Bariatric Surgery, Singapore General Hospital, Singapore, Singapore

HSIN-CHING LIN, MD, FACS
Professor and Chairman, Department of Otolaryngology, Sleep Center, Robotic Surgery Center, Kaohsiung Chang Gung Memorial Hospital, Kaohsiung City, Taiwan

STANLEY YUNG-CHUAN LIU, MD, DDS
Assistant Professor, Co-director of Sleep Surgery Fellowship, Division of Sleep Surgery, Department of Otolaryngology, Stanford University School of Medicine, Stanford, California, USA

SHAUN LOH, MBBS, MRCS (Edin), MMED (ORL)
Associate Consultant, Department of Otolaryngology, Singapore General Hospital, Singapore, Singapore

FILIPPO MONTEVECCHI, MD
Consultant, Head and Neck Department, ENT
and Oral Surgery Unit, G.B. Morgagni - L.
Pierantoni Hospital, Forlì, Italy

**JING HAO NG, BDS (Singapore), MDS
Orthodontics (Singapore), MOrth RCS
(Edinburgh, UK)**
Associate Consultant, Department of
Orthodontics, National Dental Centre,
Singapore, Singapore

**VIJAYA KRISHNAN PARAMASIVAN, MBBS,
DNB, DLO**
Consultant ENT Surgeon, Head of the
Department of Snoring and Sleep Disorders,
Madras ENT Research Foundation, Chennai,
Tamil Nadu, India

CHAN-SOON PARK, MD, PhD
Professor, Department of
Otorhinolaryngology–Head and Neck
Surgery, St Vincent's Hospital, College of
Medicine, The Catholic University of Korea,
Suwon City, Gyeonggi Province, Republic of
Korea

**CHU QIN PHUA, MBChB, MRCS (Edin),
MMED (ORL), FRCS (Edin)**
Associate Consultant, Department of
Otolaryngology, Sengkang General Hospital,
Singapore, Singapore

HSU PON POH, MBBS, MD
Head, Adjunct Professor, Department of
Otorhinolaryngology, Head and Neck Surgery,
Changi General Hospital, Singapore,
Singapore

**SHAUN RAY HAN LOH, MBBS, MRCS,
MMED (ORL)**
Otolaryngologist from Singapore, Department
of Plastic and Reconstructive Surgery, Clinical
Fellow, Craniofacial Center, Chang Gung
Memorial Hospital, Taoyuan, Taiwan;
Department of Otolaryngology, Singhealth
Duke-NUS Sleep Centre, Singapore General
Hospital, Singapore, Singapore

ROBERT RILEY, MD, DDS
Clinical Professor, Division of Sleep Surgery,
Department of Otolaryngology, Stanford
University School of Medicine, Stanford,
California, USA

SAM SHENG-PING HSU, DDS, MS
Orthodontist, Department of Plastic and
Reconstructive Surgery, Craniofacial
Center, Chang Gung Memorial Hospital,
Taoyuan, Taiwan; Esthetic Dent Clinic,
Taipei, Taiwan

CHIBA SHINTARO, MD, PhD
Professor, Department of
Otorhinolaryngology–Head and Neck Surgery,
Jikei University School of Medicine, Tokyo,
Japan

WONG HANG SIANG, MBBS, MRCP
Consultant, Department of Respiratory
and Critical Care Medicine, Changi
General Hospital, Singapore,
Singapore

**SRINIVAS KISHORE SISTLA, MBBS, MS
(ENT)**
Consultant ENT Surgeon, Head, Department of
ENT, Star Hospital, Hyderabad, Telangana,
India

SHANNON S. SULLIVAN, MD
Division of Sleep Medicine, Stanford
University, Redwood City, California, USA

**KWANG WEI THAM, MB, BCH, BAO,
ABIM**
Senior Consultant, Department of
Endocrinology, Singapore General Hospital,
Singapore, Singapore

**SONG TAR TOH, MBBS, MRCSEd,
MMED (ORL), MMED (Sleep Med),
FAMS (ORL)**
Senior Consultant, Department of
Otolaryngology, Singapore General Hospital,
Head, Singhealth Duke-NUS Sleep Centre,
Adjunct Associate Professor, National
University of Singapore, Yong Loo Lin School
of Medicine & Duke-NUS Medical School,
Singapore, Singapore

CLAUDIO VICINI, MD
Associate Professor, Otolaryngology–Head
and Neck Surgery, University of Ferrara,
Ferrara, Italy; Director, Professor, Consultant
and Head, Head and Neck Department, ENT
and Oral Surgery Unit, G.B. Morgagni - L.
Pierantoni Hospital, AUSL of Romagna, Forlì,
Italy

PO-FANG WANG, MD
Plastic and Reconstructive Surgeon,
Department of Plastic and Reconstructive
Surgery, Clinical Fellow, Craniofacial Center,
Craniofacial Research Center, Chang Gung
Memorial Hospital, College of Medicine, Chang
Gung University, Taoyuan, Taiwan

MOK YINGJUAN, MBBS, MRCP
Adjunct Assistant Professor, Consultant,
Department of Respiratory and Critical Care
Medicine, Changi General Hospital, Singapore,
Singapore

**MIMI YOW, BDS (Singapore), FDS RCS
(Edinburgh), MSc (London) (Orthodontics),
FAMS (Craniofacial Orthodontics)**
Head, Cleft and Craniofacial Deformity
Programme, Senior Consultant, Clinical
Associate Professor, Department of
Orthodontics, National Dental Centre,
Singapore, Singapore

Contents

A holistic approach is pertinent in managing obstructive sleep apnea (OSA). It goes beyond integrated multidisciplinary assessment and management in the hospital setting. Although clinicians should be aware of different treatment modalities and adjunctive measures, proactive management of OSA is as important. The future of OSA management lies in identifying patients at risk of developing OSA and developing strategy to prevent OSA from taking root. It involves active screening of patients with OSA and treating them and identifying patients with OSA with high risk of preventable serious morbidity and death and intervening early to prevent these from happening.

Abnormal breathing during sleep is related to intrinsic and extrinsic factors that are present early in life. Investigation of fetal development and early-in-life orofacial growth allows recognition of risk factors that lead to change in upper airway patency, which leads to abnormal upper airway resistance, abnormal inspiratory efforts, and further increase in resistance and progressive narrowing of the collapsible upper airway. Such evolution can be recognized by appropriate clinical evaluation, specific polysomnographic patterns, and orofacial imaging. Recognition of the problems should lead to appropriate treatments and prevention of obstructive sleep apnea and its comorbidities.

Evaluation of the upper airway is key for a successful surgical management. Proper evaluation can be done only with a good understanding of the anatomy and pathophysiology of the upper airway. The authors discuss surgical anatomy from a soft tissue and bony perspective in detail along with its clinical implications. The complex interaction among pharyngeal dilator tone, arousal threshold, respiratory control instability, and changes in lung volume during sleep play an important role in obstructive sleep apnea. Because all the anatomic and physiologic characteristics discussed have genetic predisposition, gene therapy may play a pivotal role in the future.

> Drug-induced sleep endoscopy is a safe and practical technique to evaluate the dynamic upper airway collapse during sleep. We review drug-induced sleep endoscopy in adults, including its indications, technique, evaluation of upper airway collapse, and clinical application. Drug-induced sleep endoscopy is useful to improve treatment options selection for patients with obstructive sleep apnea, especially for those who are unable to accept or tolerate continuous positive airway pressure therapy. Owing to a lack of standardization for drug-induced sleep endoscopy, it is difficult to compare the published literature from different sleep centers across the world.

> The role of the nose in the pathophysiology and treatment of sleep-disordered breathing (SDB) has not been fully understood and might have been underestimated. In the Staring resistor model, the nose is regarded as a passive and noncollapsible tube, but recent studies have shown that the nose might participate more in the pathophysiology of SDB as anatomic, neuromuscular, and respiratory factors than previously reported, which might imply the nose is an active noncollapsible tube. The roles of nasal treatments for OSA are not only the reduction of AHI, but also the improvement of subjective symptoms, sleep quality, and CPAP adherence.

> Although continuous positive airway pressure is the first-line and gold-standard management for obstructive sleep apnea (OSA), surgery is the only mainstream treatment without the use of a device. Palatal surgery is the paragon and core value among various sleep surgeries in treating snoring and OSA. It has transformed from radical excision to functional reconstruction. The integrated treatment of palatal surgery includes reconstruction of airway, restoration of airflow and rehabilitation of muscle.

> Surgery for obstructive sleep apnea/hypopnea syndrome (OSA) is not a substitute for continuous positive airway pressure (CPAP) but is a salvage procedure for those who failed CPAP and other conservative therapies and therefore have no other options. The hypopharyngeal/tongue base procedures for the treatment of OSA are usually challenging to most sleep surgeons. In recent years, several procedures for OSA patients with hypopharyngeal obstructions have been developed to achieve higher response rates with decreased postoperative morbidities.

> Nocturnal upper airway collapse often involves the obstruction at the tongue base. Several surgical procedures have been developed in recent years to

address this area in continuous positive airway pressure-nonadherent patients and include hyolingual advancement, tongue suture suspension, and various lingual resection techniques. Traditional tongue base resection is generally done either via a transcervical technique or transorally with an endoscope for visualization. Each of these approaches has significant potential limitations. The unsurpassed visualization, dexterity, and control provided by the Da Vinci Surgical System offer many benefits for the surgeon compared with the other technologies.

The structure and dimensions of the mandible, tongue, and hyoid complex are important variables in the pathophysiology of obstructive sleep apnea at the hypopharyngeal level. Genioglossus advancement is based on mandibular osteotomy, which brings the genioglossus muscle (GGM) forward and prevents posterior collapse during sleep. The genioglossus advancement technique has recently undergone several modifications; each has attempted to minimize surgical morbidity while improving the incorporation and advancement of the GGM. The hyoid bone has been of interest in sleep apnea and apnea-related surgical procedures because of its integral relationship with the tongue base and hypopharynx. Hyothyroidopexy is illustrated.

Obstructive sleep apnea is a medical syndrome with multifactorial pathophysiology. Surgery can be the primary treatment option when anatomic factors are identified with narrowing at specific or general levels of pharyngeal airway. The surgeries are directed to the etiologic anatomic structure to achieve greatest effectiveness. Body weight, Mallampati scale, and tonsil grade are key evaluations to select effective surgical procedures. Surgical weight reduction, maxillomandibular advancement, and pharyngeal soft tissue surgeries are considered for the patient with obesity, maxillomandibular retrognathism, and tonsillar hypertrophy, respectively. Tailored surgical planning can meet the patients needs for airway, esthetics, and normal Angle's occlusion.

Upper airway stimulation is a novel therapy for patients suffering from obstructive sleep apnea who are incompliant toward continuous positive airway pressure therapy. Evidence supporting the effectiveness of this therapy with regard to the treatment of disordered breathing, subjective daytime impairment, and its effect on sleep characteristics has increased. Information on the subjective sensation of the stimulation of the hypoglossal nerve could be gathered as more patients are implanted and knowledge of different aspects of the therapy is increasing. Comparisons between upper airway stimulation therapy and other surgical treatment options have been conducted. The surgical technique could be further optimized.

Whereas the original Stanford protocol relied on a tiered approach to care to avoid unnecessary surgery, it did not address the issue of surgical relapse, a common concern among sleep medicine specialists. With 3 decades of experience since the original 2-tiered Powell-Riley protocol was introduced and the role of evolving skeletal techniques and upper airway stimulation, we are pleased to present our current protocol. This update includes emphasis on the facial skeletal development with impact on function including nasal breathing, and the incorporation of upper airway stimulation. The increased versatility of palatopharyngoplasty as an adjunctive procedure is also discussed.

Obstructive sleep apnea (OSA) is a multifactorial condition, and an interdisciplinary approach to diagnosis forms the basis for effective treatment planning. Craniofacial structure and attached soft tissues and muscles play a central role in OSA. Evidence-based studies demonstrate the effectiveness of oral appliances for mandibular advancement and tongue stabilization in managing OSA, and current clinical standards of practice recommend the use of oral appliances to treat OSA when patients cannot tolerate continuous positive airway pressure (CPAP). Although effective, oral appliances are less predictable in managing OSA compared with CPAP therapy. Measures can be taken to improve predictability of oral appliance treatment.

Positional therapy appears to be an attractive strategy for many patients with positional obstructive sleep apnea (OSA). However, under the American Academy of Sleep Medicine OSA guidelines, positional therapy is considered as only an alternative therapy, because previous research has demonstrated poor treatment tolerance and adherence. Recent technological advances have renewed interest in positional therapy, with the invention of new sophisticated vibratory positional therapy devices. These devices have shown great promise with efficacy, markedly improved patient tolerance, and long-term adherence. We review the literature on positional therapy and explore the most current evidence on the new positional therapy devices.

Myofunctional therapy (MFT) has been reported to be an alternative treatment to obstructive sleep apnea (OSA), but compliance and long-term outcome in the children were considered as an issue. A prospective study was performed on age-matched children submitted to MFT or to a functional oral device used during sleep (passive MFT) and compared with no-treatment control group. Compliance is a major problem of MFT, and MFT will have to take into consideration the absolute need to have continuous parental involvement in the procedure for pediatric OSA.

Obesity plays a pivotal role in the pathogenesis of obstructive sleep apnea (OSA) and as an exacerbating factor of OSA. Given the interlinking relationship of obesity and OSA, treatment of obesity is fundamental in the management of OSA. Weight loss of 7% to 11% significantly improves OSA with remission seen with greater weight loss. Weight loss also ameliorates the constellation of other obesity-related metabolic conditions, reducing the overall cardiovascular risk in an obese person with OSA. This article discusses specific weight loss interventions effective in improving OSA, including lifestyle interventions with dietary modification and physical activity, pharmacotherapy, and bariatric surgery.

Preface

Prevention, Screening, and Treatments for Obstructive Sleep Apnea: Beyond Positive Airway Pressure (PAP)

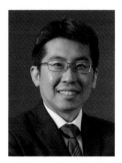

Song Tar Toh, MBBS, MRCSEd, MMED (ORL), MMED
(Sleep Med), FAMS (ORL)
Editor

The description of obstructive sleep apnea (OSA) syndrome in the 1970s was followed by the first wave of academic research to understand the pathophysiology of sleep-related abnormal breathing and upper airway obstruction, to determine its extent in the general population, and its many dire medical consequences and associations. This was followed quickly by the description of positive airway pressure (PAP) in 1981 to treat it and a second wave of academic research describing various single-modality treatments, including surgical modifications of the upper airway, oral appliances, weight management, and myofunctional therapy.

There is no doubt that PAP is currently still the mainstay of treatment. However, further understanding of this prevalent heterogenous condition brought us to the third wave, whereby academic research data provided valuable insights to better manage this condition holistically. Different health care specialties joined this endeavor to meet the demands of this condition, whereby different therapeutic modalities are used and strategies deployed to potentially delay the progression and the development of medical consequences. It has brought to our attention the need for multidisciplinary collaborations.

As these three overlapping waves continue to build upon previous data and findings, we have to rethink the need for screening for this condition in high-risk groups and the pediatric population. We need to think of screening for potential asymptomatic medical conditions associated with OSA with the aim of preventing death by treating some of these serious medical conditions associated with it.

The complex relationships between genetic predisposition and susceptibility, environmental influence, obesity, nasal respiration, craniofacial growth, intrapharyngeal airway structures, control of respiration and sleep provide fresh perspectives on how this condition can be prevented and managed.

This issue of *Sleep Medicine Clinics* dedicated to "Screening, Prevention, and Treatment of OSA: Beyond PAP" looks at some of the cutting-edge thinking behind screening and prevention strategies and increasing population awareness and utility of different non-PAP treatment for us to win the fight against this condition and its chronic medical and neurocognitive consequences.

Song Tar Toh, MBBS, MRCSEd, MMED (ORL),
MMED (Sleep Med), FAMS (ORL)
Department of Otolaryngology
Singapore General Hospital
Singhealth Duke-NUS Sleep Centre
National University of Singapore
Yong Loo Lin School of Medicine & Duke-NUS
Medical School
20 College Road, Level 5
Singapore 169856, Singapore

E-mail address:
songtar@gmail.com

Sleep Med Clin 14 (2019) xv
https://doi.org/10.1016/j.jsmc.2018.12.001
1556-407X/19/© 2018 Published by Elsevier Inc.

Holistic Management of Obstructive Sleep Apnea
Translating Academic Research to Patient Care

Song Tar Toh, MBBS, MRCSEd, MMED (ORL), MMED (Sleep Med), FAMS (ORL)[a,*],
Chu Qin Phua, MBChB, MRCS (Edin), MMED (ORL), FRCS (Edin)[b],
Shaun Loh, MBBS, MRCS (Edin), MMED (ORL)[a]

KEYWORDS
- Obstructive sleep apnea • Holistic management • Integrated approach

KEY POINTS

- Integrated multidisciplinary approach in assessment and management is important in managing patients with obstructive sleep apnea (OSA).
- Proactive management of this condition requires active screening and strategy to prevent this condition.
- The future of OSA management lies in active screening of patients at risk and for the condition, early interventions to prevent development and progression of disease, participation of patient and family physician in management process to improve outcomes and deliver cost-effective care.

INTRODUCTION
The Necessity for Holistic Management in Obstructive Sleep Apnea

Obstructive sleep apnea is a systemic disorder
Obstructive sleep apnea (OSA) is a systemic disorder, with multisystem adverse clinical associations. The numerous associations and sequelae of OSA include metabolic disturbances, cardiovascular morbidities, neurocognitive deficits, psychosocial consequences, cancer, and various other conditions (**Box 1**). OSA is also a chronic, progressive disease and if inadequately managed, can lead to multiple health care visits, increasing burden and escalating costs to health care systems around the world.

Holistic management goes beyond multidisciplinary management of this disease. It involves identifying at-risk individuals of developing this chronic condition and implementing strategy to slow or prevent its development. It involves screening for potential asymptomatic medical consequences in these patients and intervening early. It involves adjunctive measures to prevent progression of the disease and its sequelae. Engaging patients and family physician is pertinent in making OSA care more accessible and cost-effective.

Epidemiology—rising prevalence and costs of obstructive sleep apnea
OSA is a prevalent condition, with prevalence rates up to 49.7%.[1–3] Its consequential economic burden because of direct (from the diagnosis and treatment of OSA and its related

---

[a] Department of Otolaryngology, Singapore General Hospital, 20 College Road, Singapore 169856, Singapore;
[b] Department of Otolaryngology, Sengkang General Hospital, 110 Sengkang East Way, Singapore 544886, Singapore
* Corresponding author.
E-mail address: songtar@gmail.com

Sleep Med Clin 14 (2019) 1–11
https://doi.org/10.1016/j.jsmc.2018.10.014

Box 1
Known adverse associations and sequelae of obstructive sleep apnea
Metabolic
Obesity
Insulin resistance
Diabetes
Cardiovascular
Hypertension
Atherosclerosis
Ischemic heart disease
Arrhythmia
Pulmonary hypertension
Stroke
Neurologic
Dementia
Epilepsy
Depression
Poor memory
Impaired vigilance
Ophthalmology
Normal tension
Glaucoma
Floppy eyelid syndrome
Nonarteritic ischemic optic neuropathy
Urologic condition
Erectile dysfunction
Enuresis
Cancer
Increased cancer incidence
Increased cancer mortality
Psychosocial
Road traffic accidents
Impaired work productivity

sequelae such as diabetes, systemic hypertension, ischemic heart disease, and stroke) and indirect health costs (work productivity, occupational injuries as well as motor vehicle accidents) costs billions.[4–6]

It is therefore imperative that sleep physicians take an active role in screening and treating patients with OSA to reduce these costs and actively engage hospital and government policymakers to ensure resources are available to manage them.

Multimodality Management of Obstructive Sleep Apnea

OSA is a heterogeneous disorder. The pathophysiology leading to upper airway collapse and how each patient responds to airway obstruction and oxygen desaturation differs from one to another. Central to current understanding of OSA is an at-risk, compromised upper airway anatomy. Each patient with OSA has individual phenotypes by which their upper airway obstruction occurs as a complex interplay between anatomic and nonanatomic upper airway factors,[7,8] which include the following:

- At-risk upper airway anatomy
- Pharyngeal critical closure pressure
- Individual arousal threshold
- Stability of ventilatory loop gain
- Upper airway dilator muscle function
- Nocturnal rostral fluid shift
- Obesity

With this current phenotypic understanding, previous one treatment–only modality for OSA is flawed. Multimodality approach to management is thus far more effective in dealing with the multifactorial contributing factors in OSA.

These treatment strategies should be used in combination including the following:

- Weight loss and maintenance
- Sleep hygiene and lifestyle modification
- Myofunctional therapy
- Dental appliance
- Continuous positive airway pressure (CPAP)
- Surgical treatment
- Treatment of OSA according to phenotypes

Weight loss and maintenance

Patients with OSA have increased parapharyngeal fat pad volumes[9] and fat deposition in the tongue,[10] predisposing them to a narrowed upper airway. Weight loss and maintenance is important in the lifelong treatment for OSA. Peppard and colleagues[11] demonstrated that weight reduction of 10% can lead to 20% reduction of Apnea-Hypopnea Index (AHI). In addition, weight loss can potentially halt development of cardiometabolic disorders associated with OSA.[12] General weight loss advice and referral to a specialized center with expertise in medical and surgical strategies will help OSA management.

Sleep hygiene and lifestyle modification

Sleep hygiene education has been shown to improve sleep difficulties amongst patients with

OSA.[13] Optimizing sleep hygiene is essential in improving sleep quality and overall quality of life in patients with OSA and should be taught actively to them.

Sleep hygiene education involves pinpointing causation of sleep disturbance, correction of misconceptions or preformed ideas on sleep, and ensuring optimal daily habit and sleep environment to improve quality of sleep. Ideal sleep hygiene habits include: maintaining regular daily sleep schedule; ensuring comfortable sleep environment with low noise level and cool temperature; avoiding distractions in bedroom; and avoiding alcohol, nicotine, heavy meals, and caffeine before bed.

Myofunctional therapy

Myofunctional therapy targets the upper airway dilator muscles function pathway in the pathophysiology of OSA. It involves a set of exercises for the lip, tongue, soft palate, and lateral pharyngeal wall, aimed at training the upper airway dilator muscles to maintain the patency of upper airway during sleep.[14] It is hypothesized that this set of exercises increase oral and oropharyngeal muscle tone, as well as reduce fatty deposition within the tongue, thereby reducing upper airway collapsibility. Systematic review and meta-analysis by Camacho and colleagues[15] in 2015 demonstrated a statistically significant reduction of AHI from a mean of 24.5 to 12.3 per hour ($P<.0001$). In addition, improvement of lowest oxygen saturations, snoring, and sleepiness scale has also been shown.[15] These exercises can be performed in addition to other treatment modalities.

Dental appliance

Dental appliance can be used as the sole treatment or as an adjunct in the armamentarium of OSA management strategies. It reduces upper airway obstruction via advancement of the mandible, which increases lateral expansion of airway space and leads to anterior tongue movement.

It is a useful alternative, demonstrating better compliance compared with CPAP. Dental appliances have a particular role in treatment of mild to moderate OSA or as a device useful for patients with severe OSA who are unable to tolerate CPAP.[16] Furthermore, dental appliances have been shown to improve quality of life and reduce OSA-associated complications such as hypertension.[16] In patients with residual tongue obstruction after surgical modification of the airway, dental appliance can be added to achieve the desired outcome.

Treatment of obstructive sleep apnea by phenotypes

Novel concepts on pathophysiology have shed light on the complex causation of OSA. While patients with abnormal upper airway anatomy can benefit from surgical modification, patients with other endotypes such as low arousal threshold can benefit from sedatives to improve sleep quality and reduce AHI. Patients with ventilatory control instability can improve with oxygen therapy and acetazolamide, whereas patients with overnight rostral fluid shift causing OSA can benefit from diuretics, compression stockings, and head elevation.[7] Research are underway to see how these strategies can help personalize OSA treatment.

Holistic Management of Obstructive Sleep Apnea—Beyond Diagnosis and Treatment

Most of the current OSA care frameworks focus on diagnosis and treatment of the condition itself. The most typical OSA patient journey consists of attendance to General Practitioner, Otolaryngologist, Respiratory Physician, Neurologist, Dental Specialist, and Sleep Physician, with a diagnostic sleep test organized and typically standstills at referral and follow-up for treatment of OSA itself.

With the backing of academic research, the care of patient with OSA must extend beyond these consults to create a holistic OSA care system. It involves being more comprehensive and collaborative and preemptive in the management of the condition and associated comorbidities (**Fig. 1**).

Holistic management of OSA should entail the following (see **Fig. 1**):

1. Screening for associated asymptomatic comorbidities in high-risk groups and prevention of the progression of OSA-related complications, as well as continued engagement of nonsleep physicians in other specialties to increase awareness, in addition to multidisciplinary care
2. Patient-centered care and engagement
3. Screening for OSA family members
4. Engaging family physician in the OSA care
5. Identifying at-risk individual and prevention of OSA development

Screening and prevention of obstructive sleep apnea–related complications

Many epidemiologic research and publications have shown that OSA is related to many medical consequences.

This section summarizes some of the more pertinent conditions and evidence for screening and early interventions. Management of OSA should include identifying patients who are

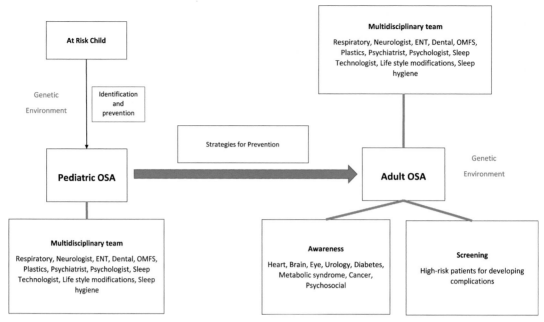

Fig. 1. Holistic OSA care system.

asymptomatic of coronary or cerebrovascular disease but at high risk of developing serious morbidity or death and intervene accordingly. Although no definite guidelines are present for some conditions at present, some researches point toward referring patients for screening. Constant engagement of other specialties to educate them on the established and emerging relationships between OSA and individual conditions will allow these conditions to be better treated, which include the following:

- Endocrinologists
- Cardiologists
- Neurologists
- Ophthalmologists
- Urologists
- Oncologists

Metabolic disturbances—obesity

Prevalence and relevance Prevalence of OSA in obese patient can range up to 80%.[17–20] Obesity and OSA have a bidirectional causal-effect relationship. Obesity is an established risk factor for OSA development and progression in multiple epidemiologic studies.[3,18,19,21] Yet OSA itself can lead to increased risks of weight gain and obesity. The pathophysiologic relationships between obesity, leptin, lung function, oxygen desaturations, appetite, and OSA are well described.[12,22,23]

At-risk patients The Wisconsin Sleep Cohort Study showed that changes in AHI correlates to weight change in a dose-response fashion.[11] The same study showed that 10% weight gain leads to 6x increased odds of developing moderate to severe OSA, independent of confounders such as age or baseline body mass index (BMI).[11] The effect of weight change on OSA severity is more marked in male patients with OSA, where a 10 kg weight gain leads to 5 times increased risk of moderate to severe OSA compared with female patients' risks of 2.5 times.[18] However, it has been shown that effect of BMI on OSA attenuates after age 60 years.[17,19]

Intervention strategies Weight management (medical and surgical strategies) should be incorporated in the overall multimodality treatment of OSA. Peppard and colleagues[11] demonstrated that weight loss of 10% can lead to 26% reduction in AHI and weight loss of 20% can lead to AHI reduction of 48%. Studies have shown that presence of intervention yields better outcome than those who did not receive help.[24] Weight loss has significant impact in reducing OSA symptoms and severity, as well as a positive effect on cholesterol levels, insulin resistance, leptin, and endothelial dysfunction.[12]

Metabolic disturbances—diabetes

Prevalence and relevance Diabetes and OSA share common risk factors such as obesity and age. Type II DM also has a two-way causal-effect relationship with OSA. Studies have showed that OSA can lead to increased incidence of insulin resistance and impaired glucose tolerance. Conversely, type II DM population has also been shown to have high prevalence of OSA. Based on findings of the Sleep Heart Health Study (USA, 2003)[25] and Sleep AHEAD study (USA, 2009),[26] the prevalence of diagnosis of OSA in type 2 diabetic patients ranges from 58% to 86%,[27] with a large proportion of type 2 diabetic individuals remaining undiagnosed.[28] The International Diabetes Federation has called for patients with type 2 diabetes to be screened for OSA and vice versa.

Postulated pathophysiologic basis of how OSA leads to diabetes mellitus stems from effect of intermittent hypoxia and sleep fragmentation, which can cause increased oxidative stress and sympathetic drive, leading to chronic low-grade systemic inflammation resulting in derangement of glucose metabolism, impairment of pancreatic beta cells, adipose tissue function, and glucose homeostasis through impaired insulin sensitivity.[29,30]

At-risk patients Patients with moderate to severe OSA are at greater risk of diabetes, with a relative risk of 1.63 compared with patients without OSA.[31]

Intervention strategies Diagnostic tests including HbA1C, fasting glucose, and glucose intolerance test can be offered to at-risk patients with OSA. Referral to endocrinologist and diabetic nurse educator for further assessment, management and education is warranted if the patients are diagnosed with type II DM. Ensuring treatment adherence to CPAP have also been proved in recent meta-analyses to help improve insulin sensitivity and glycemic control.[32,33]

Cardiovascular disease
Prevalence and relevance The Wisconsin Sleep Cohort Study demonstrated OSA to be an independent risk factor for development of hypertension.[34] The same study showed that patients with moderate OSA are at 2.89 times odds ratio of developing hypertension.[34] The Sleep Heart Health Study showed that patients with OSA have an odds ratio of 2.38 for heart failure, 1.58 for stroke, and 1.27 for coronary heart disease.[35] Study on long-term outcomes of cardiovascular outcomes in men with OSA also showed a higher odds ratio (2.87) of fatal myocardial infarction and stroke in men with untreated OSA.[36]

At-risk patients Referral to cardiology is warranted in patients with arrhythmia detected in polysomnography. Apart from that, current recommendations for cardiology screening in OSA are limited. Based on studies such as the Sleep Heart

Health Study demonstrating increased prevalence with increased AHI[35] and long-term study (mean follow-up of 10 years) by Marin and colleagues[36] showing increased fatal and nonfatal cardiovascular episodes in patients with untreated severe OSA, it would suggest that patients with severe OSA should also be referred for cardiology review. In addition, patients with concomitant comorbidities that predispose to cardiovascular conditions (eg, hypertension, hyperlipidemia) can be considered for cardiology referral.

Intervention strategies At present, treatment with CPAP as well as cardiovascular risk modification is the mainstay of reducing cardiovascular consequences of OSA. Evidence from meta-analysis demonstrated reduction of blood pressure with CPAP use.[37] Reduction of blood pressure has downstream effect of reducing cardiovascular events.[38] However, CPAP is less effective in lowering blood pressure compared with antihypertensive. Hence, combined treatment of CPAP and antihypertensive may be required for some patients with OSA with hypertension.[39]

Although observational data showed CPAP treatment reduces the risks of fatal and nonfatal cardiovascular events[36] and a prospective randomized clinical trials showed that noncompliance of CPAP therapy did not prevent cardiovascular events (SAVE),[40] a recent meta-analysis by Yu and colleagues[41] have yet to show conclusive evidence in reduction of major cardiovascular events with CPAP use.

Further studies will help delineate criteria in identifying patients with significant asymptomatic cardiovascular disease to help clinicians make referral to cardiologists for early detection and interventions.

Neurologic disorders
Prevalence and relevance Patients with OSA suffer commonly from neurocognitive impairment. These include attention deficit, poor vigilance, impaired memory, reduced visuospatial and constructional abilities, as well as poor executive functions (including volition, planning, purposeful actions).[42–44] Neurologic disorders linked to OSA include stroke, epilepsy, neurodegenerative disease, Alzheimer, Parkinson disease, and multisystem atrophy.[45]

At-risk patients OSA severity by AHI criteria,[12] hypoxaemia,[46] and sleep fragmentation[44] have been shown in some studies to cause the development of the neurocognitive disorders. However, this is not fully conclusive. It remains a clinical conundrum on when we should screen OSA who are deemed to be at-risk patients for stroke. It also remains to be discussed how proactive clinicians should be in referring such cases to neurologist for active management.

Intervention strategies There are currently no guidelines regarding when to refer patients to neurologist for evaluation regarding stroke risk in patients with OSA. Further research into this area is needed to help provide guidance for the Sleep community.

Ophthalmic conditions
Prevalence and relevance One of the most commonly reported ophthalmic sequelae of OSA is glaucoma. Prevalence of glaucoma in patients with OSA ranges from 3% to 27%.[47] Patients with OSA have a hazard ratio of 1.88 in developing glaucoma compared with normal controls.[48] Other ophthalmic conditions associated with OSA include floppy eyelid syndrome, nonarteritic anterior optic neuropathy, papilloedema, retinal vein occlusion, age-related macular degeneration, and central serous retinopathy.[49–52] Pathophysiologic hypotheses behind ocular injury from OSA includes intermittent hypoxia causing damage to optic nerve head and retinal ganglion cells, as well as vascular dysregulation leading to poor ocular perfusion and raised intraocular pressure.[47] Ocular injury can also occur from treatment of OSA with CPAP.

At-risk patients Risk factors for developing glaucoma or disease progression includes increased OSA severity,[53] untreated OSA,[48] increased age,[54] and increased BMI.[54]

Intervention strategies Referral to ophthalmologist for a thorough evaluation should be performed for all patients with OSA, given the risks and prevalence of glaucoma. This is of particular relevance, especially given that CPAP treatment can increase intraocular pressure and thereby predispose patients to worsening glaucoma.[55] While on CPAP treatment, regular intraocular pressuring monitoring may need to be performed to monitor for glaucoma development and eye damage.

Urology
Prevalence and relevance Urologic conditions associated with OSA include nocturia, enuresis, erectile dysfunction, and overactive bladder. Prevalence of nocturia in patients with OSA was reported to be up to 47.8%.[56] Prevalence of erectile dysfunction in patients with OSA has been reported to be as high as 69%.[57]

At-risk patients Nocturia and nocturnal enuresis has been shown to be associated with age and OSA severity.[58,59] Predictors of worse erectile dysfunction include increasing age and concurrent diabetes.[60]

Intervention strategies Screening of urologic symptoms should be part of the systemic history taking for patients with OSA. Urologists should be cognizant of association of lower urinary tract symptoms with OSA and active referral to sleep physicians for at-risk patients.

Cancer
Prevalence and relevance There is an association of increased cancer incidence (pancreatic, renal, melanoma),[61] progression,[62] aggressiveness,[62] and mortality[63] with OSA.

At-risk patients Patients with OSA at risk of higher cancer incidence and poorer prognosis include younger patients, severe OSA, untreated OSA, male sex, nonobese patients, patients with other sleep disorders, and patients without excessive daytime sleepiness.[62] Lower oxygen saturations, patients younger than 45 years, and severe OSA have been shown to have higher all-type cancer incidence and incidence of cancer mortality.[63–66]

Intervention strategies The effect of OSA treatment on reducing cancer incidence and mortality is yet to be fully established, but CPAP treatment may confer some protection against cancer development and progression.[64,67]

Screening for family members with obstructive sleep apnea and in pediatrics population
Previous studies have shown familial aggregation of OSA.[68,69] The Cleveland Family study, one of the largest family-based studies on sleep apnea showed that sleep-disordered breathing was more prevalent in the relatives of patients with confirmed diagnosis of sleep-disordered breathing.[69] The heritability of OSA can be explained in part by inheritance of common risk factors for OSA, including obesity and craniofacial morphologies.

Although at present there is insufficient evidence to justify the benefits of screening of OSA in asymptomatic populations,[70] given the disease burden and potential sequelae, it may be useful to consider screening family members during health maintenance evaluations. Useful screening questionnaires include the Berlin Questionnaire, STOP-BANG questionnaire (Snoring, Tiredness, Observed apnea, high blood Pressure, BMI, Age, Neck circumference, Gender), Multivariable apnea prediction score, and the Wisconsin Sleep Questionnaire.

The American Academy of Pediatrics recommended screening all children and adolescents for symptoms of snoring and OSA, during routine health visits.[71] This can be followed by more detailed assessment by sleep specialists. Treatments of pediatrics OSA using single modality often fails to eliminate it completely, setting the stage for development of adult OSA. Hence multimodality treatment and finding appropriate strategy to continue to manage these patients may help prevent OSA from developing in some patient groups (see **Fig. 1**).

Patient-centered care and patient engagement
Traditional model of care involves referral of the patient with OSA from primary care physician to individual specialists, which often leads to multiple appointments, repetition of evaluations and tests, prolonged wait time to treatment, and lack of coordinated care. This fragmented care is often non–cost-effective and unsatisfactory for patients.

There is a current paradigm shift toward patient-centered care, which can involve a creation of a clinical care surrounding the patient. It involves the primary physician, sleep center, use of telemedicine, and educating and understanding the patients to allow shared management of this chronic condition (**Fig. 2**).

In the setting of OSA, it involves creation of multidisciplinary network around the patient, involving the Sleep technologist, Dietician, Physiotherapist, Nurse Educator, Primary Care Physician, ENT Surgeon, Respiratory Physician, Dentist, Oral Maxillofacial Surgeon, Psychologist and Psychiatrist. Creation of multidisciplinary sleep center enables a team-based approach to patient's condition and enables the application of breadth and depth of various expertise to deal with diagnostic and therapeutic challenges.

Patient-centered care also involves considering the patient's needs, and expectations are considered when tailoring treatment for their OSA. Systematic review on patient-centered care showed a positive impact on patient satisfaction and self-management.[72] Different patient will have different motivation for seeking treatment in OSA. Patient-centered outcomes should therefore be the priority when patient is treated for OSA. The top 6 outcomes patients are concerned with include the following[73]:

- Prevention of long-term complications of sleep disorders
- Improve daytime functioning
- Reduce mortality
- Improve general health
- Promote treatment adherence
- Improve sleep symptoms

With regard to factors affecting treatment choices for OSA, patients are concerned about the following[74]:

- Device effectiveness
- Transportability
- Embarrassment of using the treatment
- Cost

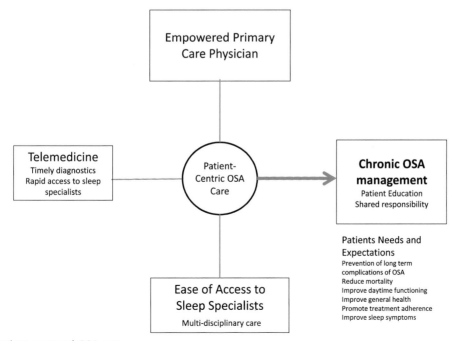

Fig. 2. Patient-centered OSA care.

In working toward a shared decision-making in OSA management, intervention offered should consider how treatment fits within the context of the patient's daily life. Support should be given to help patients integrate the management of their condition with the patients' activities of daily living. For instance, a CPAP user, who is also a frequent business traveler, should be given a doctor's letter to ease travel.

Advancement of technology can be harnessed to facilitate patient-centered care. Development of ambulatory sleep diagnostic devices allows diagnosis of OSA in the comfort of the patient's own home, eliminating the first-night effect, as well as solving the problem of huge clinical demand.[1–3,75]

Telemedicine and electronic messaging remove the barrier of distance travel and allow rapid access to information and specialist consult. Telemedicine has been shown to have positive impact on CPAP adherence.[76] Cloud-based storage of CPAP therapy data can increase the responsiveness of health care professional in patient care by allowing real-time monitoring and intervention remotely.

Patients' health seeking behavior is also tied to their health beliefs. In particular, the perceived severity and implications of a condition can affect the patient's motivation for treatment.[77] Patient education hence plays a big role in modifying this behavior. The ultimate aim would be to align the understanding of the disease process, condition severity, impact on quality of life, and treatment goal between the patient and health care team.

Patient engagement encourages ownership and is paramount in the management of chronic illnesses such as OSA. Fostering this spirit of patient empowerment encourages shared responsibility in maintenance of patient's health. Education regarding care of their condition and treatment should be performed to equip patients with the ability to self-manage their condition in their daily lives. Individualizing treatment target can be done, with active involvement of the patient in the decision-making.

Engaging family physician in the treatment of these patients

Engagement and involvement of primary care physician in the overall care of the patients with OSA is also of equal importance. In the delivery of patient-centered care, primary care physicians offer the valuable role of accessibility and are the constant point of care. It expands OSA care beyond the limited tertiary care centers, to the more widely accessible primary care network.

Given the multiple associated comorbidities of OSA, primary care physicians play a pivotal role in coordinating the management of the patient's OSA and comorbidities. With adequate training and support, the primary care physician can offer initial diagnosis and evaluation of the patients with OSA, provide annual check-up for a stable patient with OSA, and refer on to subspecialists should any issues arise. Chai-Coetzer and colleagues[78] showed that primary care management of OSA was equivalent to that of a specialist sleep center in reduction of symptoms, treatment adherence, and patient satisfaction (see **Fig. 2**).

Prevention of OSA development

Recent insights and understanding of OSA refreshed the authors' perspectives. Current management paradigm focus on prevention of OSA and details can be found in Christian Guilleminault and colleagues', "Sleep-Disordered-Breathing, Orofacial Growth and Prevention of Obstructive Sleep Apnea", in this issue. Their understanding of pathophysiology of OSA, nasal respiration, use of tongue, and craniofacial skeletal and soft tissue development offers an exciting avenue to explore strategies in preventing OSA and its associated morbidities and mortality.

SUMMARY

OSA is global health epidemic and the sleep physician has a heavy responsibility to shoulder. Proactive and holistic approach is pivotal in preventing and treating this disease, containing this growing disease burden that leads to disability and death. Integrated approach using patient-centered care line, screening and prevention of complications, as well as patient education and engagement are essential in ensuring successful intervention and optimized patient outcomes.

REFERENCES

1. Bixler EO, Vgontzas AN, Ten Have T, et al. Effects of age on sleep apnea in men: I. Prevalence and severity. Am J Respir Crit Care Med 1998;157: 144–8 [PubMed].
2. Bixler EO, Vgontzas AN, Lin HM, et al. Prevalence of sleep-disordered breathing in women: effects of gender. Am J Respir Crit Care Med 2001;163(3 Pt 1):608–13.
3. Heinzer R, Vat S, Marques-Vidal P, et al. Prevalence of sleep-disordered breathing in the general population: the HypnoLaus study. Lancet Respir Med 2015; 3:310–8.
4. Frost, Sullivan. Hidden health crisis costing America billions. Underdiagnosing and undertreating obstructive sleep apnea draining healthcare system.

Darien (IL): American Academy of Sleep Medicine; 2016. Available at: http://www.aasmnet.org/sleep-apnea-economic-impact.aspx.

5. Sherman B. Obstructive sleep apnea and health benefits purchasing: an employer perspective. J Clin Sleep Med 2013;9:187–9.

6. Sassani A, Findley LJ, Kryger M, et al. Reducing motor-vehicle collisions, costs, and fatalities by treating obstructive sleep apnea syndrome. Sleep 2004;27:453–8.

7. Subramani Y, Singh M, Wong J, et al. Understanding phenotypes of obstructive sleep apnea: applications in anesthesia, surgery, and perioperative medicine. Anesth Analg 2017;124(1):179–91.

8. Eckert DJ, White DP, Jordan AS, et al. Defining phenotypic causes of obstructive sleep apnea. Identification of novel therapeutic targets. Am J Respir Crit Care Med 2013;188(8):996–1004.

9. Li Y, Lin N, Ye J, et al. Upper airway fat tissue distribution in subjects with obstructive sleep apnea and its effect on retropalatal mechanical loads. Respir Care 2012;57(7):1098–105.

10. Kim AM, Keenan BT, Jackson N, et al. Tongue fat and its relationship to obstructive sleep apnea. Sleep 2014;37(10):1639–48.

11. Peppard PE, Young T, Palta M, et al. Longitudinal study of moderate weight change and sleep-disordered breathing. JAMA 2000;284(23):3015–21.

12. Romero-Corral A, Caples SM, Lopez-Jimenez F, et al. Interactions between obesity and obstructive sleep apnea. Chest 2010;137(1):711–9.

13. Guedes Bahia M, Soares V, Carlos Winkck J. Impact of sleep hygiene on patients with obstructive sleep apnoea syndrome. Rev Port Pneumol 2006;12(2): 147–76.

14. Guimaraes KC, Drager LF, Genta PR, et al. Effects of oropharyngeal exercises on patients with moderate obstructive sleep apnea syndrome. Am J Respir Crit Care Med 2009;179:962–6.

15. Camacho M, Certal V, Abdullatif J, et al. Myofunctional therapy to treat obstructive sleep apnea: a systematic review and meta-analysis. Sleep 2015; 38(5):669–75.

16. Ramar K, Dort LC, Katz SG, et al. Clinical practice guideline for the treatment of obstructive sleep apnea and snoring with oral appliance therapy: an update for 2015. J Clin Sleep Med 2015;11(7): 773–827.

17. Young T, Peppard PE, Taheri S. Excess weight and sleep disordered breathing. J Appl Physiol (1985) 2005;99(4):1592–9.

18. Newman AB, Foster G, Givelber R, et al. Progression and regression of sleep-disordered breathing with changes in weight: the Sleep Heart Health Study. Arch Intern Med 2005;165(20):2408–13.

19. Tishler PV, Larkin EK, Schluchter MD, et al. Incidence of sleep-disordered breathing in an urban adult population: the relative importance of risk factors in the development of sleep-disordered breathing. JAMA 2003;289:2230–7.

20. Povitz M, James MT, Pendharkar SR, et al. Prevalence of sleep-disordered breathing in obese patients with chronic hypoxemia. a cross-sectional study. Ann Am Thorac Soc 2015;12(6):921–7.

21. Peppard PE, Young T, Barnet JH, et al. Increased prevalence of sleep disordered breathing in adults. Am J Epidemiol 2013;177:1006–14.

22. Schwartz AR, Patil SP, Laffan AM, et al. Obesity and obstructive sleep apnea - pathogenic mechanisms and therapeutic approaches. Proc Am Thorac Soc 2008;5(2):185–92.

23. Joosten SA, Hamilton GS, Naughton MT. Impact of weight loss management in OSA. Chest 2017; 152(1):194–203.

24. Tuomilehto HP, Seppä JM, Partinen MM, et al. Kuopio Sleep Apnea Group Lifestyle intervention with weight reduction: first-line treatment in mild obstructive sleep apnea. Am J Respir Crit Care Med 2009; 179(4):320–7.

25. Resnick HE, Redline S, Shahar E, et al. Diabetes and sleep disturbances: findings from the Sleep Heart Health Study. Diabetes Care 2003;26:702–9.

26. Foster GD, Sanders MH, Millman R, et al. Obstructive sleep apnea among obese patients with type 2 diabetes. Diabetes Care 2009;32:1017–9.

27. Pamidi S, Tasali E. Obstructive sleep apnea and type 2 diabetes: is there a link? Front Neurol 2012;3:126.

28. Heffner JE, Rozenfeld Y, Kai M, et al. Prevalence of diagnosed sleep apnea among patients with type 2 diabetes in primary care. Chest 2012;141:1414–21.

29. Nannapeneni S, Ramar K, Surani S. Effect of obstructive sleep apnea on type 2 diabetes mellitus: a comprehensive literature review. World J Diabetes 2013;4(6):238–44.

30. Clarenbach CF, West SD, Kohleh M. Is obstructive sleep apnea a risk factor for diabetes. Discov Med 2011;12(62):17–24.

31. Wang X, Bi Y, Zhang Q, et al. Obstructive sleep apnoea and the risk of type 2 diabetes: a meta-analysis of prospective cohort studies. Respirology 2013;18:140–6.

32. Iftikhar IH, Khan MF, Das A, et al. Meta-analysis: continuous positive airway pressure improves insulin resistance in patients with sleep apnea without diabetes. Ann Am Thorac Soc 2013;10:115–20.

33. Yang D, Liu Z, Yang H, et al. Effects of continuous positive airway pressure on glycemic control and insulin resistance in patients with obstructive sleep apnea: a meta-analysis. Sleep Breath 2013;17: 33–8.

34. Peppard PE, Young T, Palta M, et al. Prospective study of the association between sleep-disordered breathing and hypertension. N Engl J Med 2000; 342(19):1378–84.

35. Shahar E, Whitney CW, Redline S, et al. Sleep-disordered breathing and cardiovascular disease: cross-sectional results of the Sleep Heart Health Study. Am J Respir Crit Care Med 2001;163(1): 19–25.

36. Marin JM, Carrizo SJ, Vicente E, et al. Long-term cardiovascular outcomes in men with obstructive sleep apnoea– hypopnoea with or without treatment with continuous positive airway pressure: an observational study. Lancet 2005;365(9464): 1046–53.

37. Haentjens P, Van Meerhaeghe A, Moscariello A, et al. The impact of continuous positive airway pressure on blood pressure in patients with obstructive sleep apnea syndrome: evidence from a meta-analysis of placebo-controlled randomized trials. Arch Intern Med 2007;167(8):757.

38. Turnbull F, Blood Pressure Lowering Treatment Trialists' Collaboration. Effects of different blood-pressure-lowering regimens on major cardiovascular events: results of prospectively-designed overviews of randomised trials. Lancet 2003;362(9395): 1527–35.

39. Pépin JL, Tamisier R, Barone-Rochette G, et al. Comparison of continuous positive airway pressure and valsartan in hypertensive patients with sleep apnea. Am J Respir Crit Care Med 2010;182(7):954.

40. McEvoy RD, Antic NA, Heeley E, et al, SAVE Investigators and Coordinators. CPAP for prevention of cardiovascular events in obstructive sleep apnea. N Engl J Med 2016;375(10):919.

41. Yu J, Zhou Z, McEvoy RD, et al. Association of positive airway pressure with cardiovascular events and death in adults with sleep apnea: a systematic review and meta-analysis. JAMA 2017;318(2):156.

42. Engleman HM, Kingshott RN, Martin SE, et al. Cognitive function in the sleepapnea/hypopnea syndrome (SAHS). Sleep 2000;23:S102–8.

43. Beebe DW, Groesz L, Wells C, et al. The neuropsychological effects of obstructive sleep apnea: a meta-analysis of norm-referenced and case-controlled data. Sleep 2003;26:298–307.

44. Bucks RS, Olaithe M, Eastwood P. Neurocognitive function in obstructive sleep apnea: a meta-review. Respirology 2013;18:61–70.

45. Ferini-Strambi L, Lombardi GE, Marelli S, et al. Neurological deficits in obstructive sleep apnea. Curr Treat Options Neurol 2017;19:16.

46. Aloia MS, Arnedt JT, Davis JD, et al. Neuropsychological sequelae of obstructive sleep apnea-hypopnea syndrome: a critical review. J Int Neuropsychol Soc 2004;10(5):772–85.

47. Chaitanya A, Pai VH, Mohapatra AK, et al. Glaucoma and its association with obstructive sleep apnea: a narrative review. Oman J Ophthalmol 2016; 9(3):125–34.

48. Chen HY, Chang YC, Lin CC, et al. Obstructive sleep apnea patients having surgery are less associated with glaucoma. J Ophthalmol 2014; 2014:838912.

49. Pérez-Rico C, Gutiérrez-Díaz E, Mencía-Gutiérrez E, et al. Obstructive sleep apnea-hypopnea syndrome (OSAHS) and glaucomatous optic neuropathy. Graefes Arch Clin Exp Ophthalmol 2014;252: 1345–57.

50. McNab AA. The eye and sleep. Clin Exp Ophthalmol 2005;33:117–25.

51. Khurana RN, Porco TC, Claman DM, et al. Increasing sleep duration is associated with geographic atrophy and age-related macular degeneration. Retina 2016;36:255–8.

52. Stein JD, Kim DS, Mundy KM, et al. The association between glaucomatous and other causes of optic neuropathy and sleep apnea. Am J Ophthalmol 2011;152:989–98.e3.

53. Lin PW, Friedman M, Lin HC, et al. Normal tension glaucoma in patients with obstructive sleep apnea/hypopnea syndrome. J Glaucoma 2011; 20:553–8.

54. Bendel RE, Kaplan J, Heckman M, et al. Prevalence of glaucoma in patients with obstructive sleep apnoea – a cross-sectional case-series. Eye (Lond) 2008;22:1105–9.

55. Kiekens S, De Groot V, Coeckelbergh T, et al. Continuous positive airway pressure therapy is associated with an increase in intraocular pressure in obstructive sleep apnea. Invest Ophthalmol Vis Sci 2008;49(3):934–40.

56. Hajduk IA, Strollo PJ Jr, Jasani RR, et al. Prevalence and predictors of nocturia in obstructive sleep apnea-hypopnea syndrome–a retrospective study. Sleep 2003;26(1):61–4.

57. Campos-Juanatey F, Fernandez- Barriales M, Gonzalez M, et al. Effects of obstructive sleep apnea and its treatment over the erectile function: a systematic review. Asian J Androl 2017;19(3): 303–10.

58. PÅ,ywaczewski R, StokÅ,osa A, Bednarek M, et al. Nocturia in obstructive sleep apnoea (OSA). Pneumonol Alergol Pol 2007;75:140–6.

59. Alexopoulos E, Malakasioti G, Varlami V, et al. Nocturnal enuresis is associated with moderate-to severe obstructive sleep apnea in children with snoring. Pediatr Res 2014;76:555–9.

60. Santos T, Drummond M, Botelho F. Erectile dysfunction in obstructive sleep apnea syndrome–prevalence and determinants. Rev Port Pneumol 2012; 18(2):64–71.

61. Subash Shantha GP, Kumar AA, Cheskin LJ, et al. Association between sleep-disordered breathing, obstructive sleep apnea, and cancer incidence: a systematic review and meta-analysis. Sleep Med 2015;16(10):1289–94.

62. Martinez-Garcia MA, Campos-Rodriguez F, Barbe F. Cancer and OSA - current evidence from human studies. Chest 2016;150(2):451–63.

63. Nieto FJ, Peppard PE, Young T, et al. Sleep-disordered breathing and cancer mortality: results from the Wisconsin Sleep Cohort Study. Am J Respir Crit Care Med 2012;186(2):190–4.

64. Campos-Rodriguez F, Martinez-Garcia MA, Martinez M, et al. Association between obstructive sleep apnea and cancer incidence in a large multicenter Spanish cohort. Am J Respir Crit Care Med 2013;187(1):99–105.

65. Gozal D, Ham SA, Mokhlesi B. Sleep apnea and cancer: analysis of a nationwide population sample. Sleep 2016;39(8):1493–500.

66. Brenner R, Kivity S, Peker M, et al. Increased risk for cancer in young patients with severe obstructive sleep apnea. Sleep 2017;40(suppl1):231.

67. Chen JC, Hwang JH. Sleep apnea increased incidence of primary central nervous system cancers: a nationwide cohort study. Sleep Med 2014;15(7):749–54.

68. Strohl KP, Saunders NA, Feldman NT, et al. Obstructive sleep apnea in family members. N Engl J Med 1978;299(18):969–73.

69. Redline S, Tishler PV, Tosteson TD, et al. The familial aggregation of obstructive sleep apnea. Am J Respir Crit Care Med 1995;151(3 Pt 1):682–7.

70. US Preventive Services Task Force. Screening for obstructive sleep apnea in adults US Preventive Services Task Force recommendation statement. JAMA 2017;317(4):407–14.

71. Marcus CL, Brooks LJ, Draper KA, et al. Diagnosis and management of childhood obstructive sleep apnea syndrome. Pediatrics 2012;130:576–84.

72. Rathert C, Wyrwich MD, Boren SA. Patient-centered care and outcomes: a systematic review of the literature. Med Care Res Rev 2013;70(4):351–79.

73. Havens C, Seixas A, Jean-Louis G, et al, Sleep Research Network. Patient and provider perspectives on patient-centered outcomes in sleep apnea. Sleep 2018;41(suppl_1):A191.

74. Almeida FR, Henrich N, Marra C, et al. Patient preferences and experiences of CPAP and oral appliances for the treatment of obstructive sleep apnea: a qualitative analysis. Sleep Breath 2013;17(2):659–66.

75. Kapur VK, Auckley DH, Chowdhuri S, et al. Clinical practice guidelines for diagnostic testing for adult sleep apnea: an American Academy of Sleep Medicine clinical practice guidelines. J Clin Sleep Med 2017;13(3):479–504.

76. Chang J, Derose S, Benjafield A, et al. Acceptance and impact of telemedicine in patient sub-groups with obstructive sleep apnea: aalysis from the tele-OSA randomized clinical trial. Sleep 2017;40(Suppl 1):A201–2.

77. Hilbert J, Yaggi HK. Patient-centered care in obstructive sleep apnea: a vision for the future. Sleep Med Rev 2018;37:138–47.

78. Chai-Coetzer CL, Antic NA, Rowland LS, et al. Primary care vs specialist sleep center management of obstructive sleep apnea and daytime sleepiness and quality of life a randomized trial. JAMA 2013;309(10):997–1004.

Sleep-Disordered Breathing, Orofacial Growth, and Prevention of Obstructive Sleep Apnea

Christian Guilleminault, DM, MD, DBiol[a],*,
Shannon S. Sullivan, MD[a], Yu-shu Huang, MD, PhD[b]

KEYWORDS

• Upper airway • Abnormal resistance • Sleep states • Orofacial growth • Prevention

KEY POINTS

• Orofacial growth is involved in factors leading to obstructive sleep apnea; untreated abnormal growth leads to upper airway resistance.
• Upper airway resistance due to abnormal orofacial growth leads to increased collapse of upper airway during sleep.
• Recognition and treatment of factors involved in abnormal orofacial growth prevent sleep-disordered breathing.

INTRODUCTION

Often, patients are not diagnosed with sleep-disordered breathing (SDB) or obstructive sleep apnea (OSA) until approximately 40 years of age. This is unfortunate because a diagnosis of SDB at this age is accompanied by various comorbidities, including excessive daytime sleepiness, increased risk of traffic, and industrial accidents and cardiovascular complications. Each year, new epidemiologic studies demonstrate associations between sleep apnea and metabolic dysfunction; psychiatric, neurologic, and ophthalmologic syndromes; and pregnancy complications. Part of the increase in the prevalence of sleep apnea can be attributed to the rising occurrence of obesity in many countries. There is a long known association between the prevalence of OSA and obesity. This phenomenon has been seen in both adults and children.[1]

The presence of OSA in children was shown, however, in 1976,[2] and the observation that OSA is familial and can be noted in both children and adults in the same families was well demonstrated in different parts of the world in the 1990s.[3,4,5] The dissociation of adult and pediatric OSA is thus completely artificial; to the contrary, the underpinnings and development of SDB follow a continuum across age. Acknowledging this longitudinal aspect has led to studies to identify what is behind SDB and what the factors are that lead to abnormal breathing during sleep.

It can be argued that the adult overweight OSA patient is at the end of the line. By this time, clinically relevant comorbidities are present, and detection of OSA at this point is already too late. The absence of education on early identification is responsible for this sad state of medical care. Elements leading to SDB should be detected much earlier; treatment should be attempted at the

None of the authors as conflict of interest.
[a] Division of Sleep Medicine, Stanford University, 450 Broadway Pavillion C 2nd Floor, Redwood City, CA 94063, USA; [b] Division of Child-Psychiatry and Pediatric-Sleep laboratory, Department of Psychiatry, Chang Gung Memorial Hospital and Medical College, No. 5, Fuxing Street, Guishan, Taoyuan 333, Linkou, Taiwan
* Corresponding author.
E-mail address: cguil@stanford.edu

Sleep Med Clin 14 (2019) 13–20
https://doi.org/10.1016/j.jsmc.2018.11.002
1556-407X/19/© 2018 Elsevier Inc. All rights reserved.

earliest recognition of problems. Efforts toward prevention should be made as early as possible, and the appropriate multidisciplinary specialists should be involved in care. It does not mean that very early recognition always leads to avoidance of the full-blown problem and that positive airway pressure [PAP] treatment will be avoided, but at least comorbidities should be avoided entirely or, in part, recognizing that compliance with any treatment is never perfect. Waiting until adulthood for otolaryngologic procedures, such as uvulopalatopharyngoplasty, has been shown on the whole to be inadequate in the long-term, complete resolution of OSA, further emphasizing the need for early, more prevention-driven therapies.

THE UPPER AIRWAY

The upper airway (UA) is a collapsible tube surrounded by muscles that are controlled by reflexes that develop during fetal life. Genetic and environmental factors have a direct impact on the development of the UA and its supports. The UA size is related to the development of its bony supports, which are controlled initially by genetic input and later on joined by environmental factors and the interaction of environmental factors on genes.

FETAL LIFE

During early fetal life,[6,7] the 39 homeobox genes have a major influence on the development of the UA region. Five modules derived from the ectoderm are responsible for the formation of face, teeth, and UA. Genetic mutations at this stage are responsible for different forms of Pierre Robin syndrome or other important malformations, such as DiGeorge and Shprintzen-Goldberg syndromes, among others. These syndromes are associated with important malformations, and one of the findings at birth is abnormal breathing during sleep. Near the tenth week of gestational age, formation of the permanent mouth begins. The tongue becomes horizontal, and primordial neuronal networks that become various cranial nerves important for UA function are formed. Resultant functions are clearly visible with fetal echography at this stage, including initiation of sucking and swallowing function using sensory-motor reflexes. Such reflexes are triggered by contact between tongue and palate and the lips and palate. In addition, contact between different parts of the body with the lips, which triggers protrusion of the tongue and suction, is followed by swallow and the initial step of the esophageal reflex. With maturation of the fetus, the Hooker reflexes that are similar to the so-

called primitive reflexes seen at birth with stimulation of lips are observed. During the last trimester of pregnancy there is a continuous training of the suck-swallow reflex with transit of 1 mL of amniotic fluid initially, which increases to approximately 500 nL just before birth.

During fetal life, training of diaphragm and respiratory accessory muscles must also occur, but of course the use of the UA for the passage of air to the lungs does not occur before birth. Instead, studies of the fetus using echography,[8] as well as of premature infants, have shown that the final 3 months of gestation are a training period for the complex activity of the UA and of reflexes needed for the vital functions of sucking and swallowing with protection of the airway. The fetus also develops clear periods of rest and activity and periods of active sleep with activation of facial muscles. Studies of premature infants have shown that active sleep (the rapid eye movement [REM] correlate) can be detected clearly in premature infants of 27 weeks' gestation, and fetal echography has also shown the presence of grimace, smile, and facial twitches indicative of active sleep. This represents a training of orofacial muscles; this activity is similar to what is observed at term birth during active sleep. Similarly, training of chest muscles occurs during repetitive occurrence of active sleep.

Studies of premature infants have shown that the more premature the infant, the more health problems are present. There is a clear impact of the absence of complete UA training with premature birth: the size of the oral cavity is abnormally small, and in addition muscles are hypotonic, in particular, those involved in UA functions and facial functions. In addition, premature infants also often present with immaturity of brainstem functions, including control of breathing, which leads to diaphragmatic apnea (central apnea) but also weakness of UA and facial muscles. The failure of normal and complete UA training and structural development has an immediate impact in the postnatal life, directly proportional to the degree of prematurity and ultimately leading to deficiencies in orofacial growth.

At birth, 2 growth centers are known to still be active: the intermaxillary synchondrosis and the alveolodental ligament.[9] Stimulation of these 2 growth centers are important for the continuation of orofacial growth in postnatal life and the further development of bone supports for the upper airway. These growth centers have been shown to be stimulated by specific behaviors occurring immediately after birth: sucking and swallowing stimulate the intermaxillary cartilage, as do nasal breathing and facial expressions. Jaw movements and pressure stimulate the alveolodental ligament. Growth in the orofacial region is due to endochondral ossification, that is, build-up of bones from a cartilaginous framework. Performing normal orofacial functions after birth provides the stimulus to further develop orofacial structures that support the UA. Any impairment in such function can have an impact both immediately and lastingly on growth. Early life is a particularly vulnerable period because orofacial growth velocity is highest between birth and 2 years of age and remains highly active until 6 years of age. By this age, 60% of the normal adult face is built. A second period of high growth velocity occurs at puberty.

Unfortunately, the clinical sequelae of early UA growth interruption or abnormality are persistent. Investigation of a large premature infant cohort has shown that SDB is noted early in the development, and follow-up studies showed that 77% of 400 premature infants have OSA at 4 years of age.[10,11] One of the conclusions from this work is that the reduction or absence of orofacial muscle training, alongside a generalized hypotonia also involving orofacial muscles, did not permit a normal orofacial development. This disturbance in normal muscle function alters structural growth, which leads to more restricted bony supports for the muscles forming the UA.

DISCRETE ANOMALIES OF OROFACIAL GROWTH

As detailed previously,[10] investigation of 2000 children and review of experimental studies performed on newborn rhesus monkeys demonstrated that 1 mechanism in particular had an impact on the orofacial growth early on: the absence of stimulation of the critical early-life UA 2 growth centers, discussed previously. This seems to be a common pathway to abnormal orofacial growth, but the upstream, underlying causes of the absence of appropriate stimulation were variable. Sources included genetic or inflammatory cartilage diseases (such as Marfan syndrome, Ehlers-Danlos syndromes, juvenile rheumatoid arthritis, and genetic absence of permanent teeth [oligodontia]), genetic muscle disorders (such as myotonic dystrophy and Duchenne dystrophy), and also mechanical UA obstruction or dysfunction (eg enlarged adenoids and tonsils, short lingual frenulum, and nasal turbinate hypertrophy, particularly due to allergies, substantial septal deviation early in life) and early dental extraction (before 12 years of age) of permanent tooth roots.[10] Each of these problems (and some that may not have been included) led to mouth breathing; abnormal position of the tongue in the mouth cavity; and

decrease or absence of the normal stimulation of the intermaxillary cartilage, the alveolodental ligament, and/or probably the mandibular condyle cartilage, the latter being less investigated. Such dysfunction occurs early in life, at a time when orofacial growth is at maximum, so consequences of suboptimal, abnormal growth may be experienced for decades. Intermediate mechanisms include the development of mouth breathing and disuse of the normal nasal breathing. The absence of the normal development of the orofacial growth also has secondary consequences on the maxillomandibular position. Such changes have a negative feedback impact on the insertion of the muscles forming the UA.

UPPER AIRWAY: A COLLAPSIBLE TUBE

The UA is formed by muscles that are controlled by different cranial nerves. Functions include sucking, swallowing, breathing, and speech— that is, very different functions, most of which involve reflexes developed before or at birth and rarely between 6 months and 12 months of age. As discussed previously, these muscles are inserted on bones that are mostly part of the orofacial structure. Investigations of UA collapsibility indicate that intrinsic and extrinsic factors are involved in maintenance of UA patency.

Both genetics and environment may play a role in intrinsic factors. First, each muscle fiber has a response to tension. Second, there is contribution from local air pressure to collapsibility of UA: during inspiration there is a short time when the UA is subjected to subatmospheric pressure. Calculation of the critical pressure (Pcrit) gave information on the relationship between closure of UA and atmospheric pressure, and these elements are considered intrinsic factors. The basic formula relating Pcrit to airflow is as follows: $Vmax = (Pn - Pcrit)/Rn$, where Pn is nasal pressure, Rn is nasal resistance, and $Vmax$ is maximum airflow. It is also known that UA is maintained open due to reflexes that specifically placed under tension different upper-airway muscles in the UA, the most important being the protrusive fibers of the tongue that are innervated by nerve fibers located at the distal aspects of the XII nerve. These reflexes can be impacted by injuries to the sensory-motor loop, altering tension of the muscle during inspiration, but these reflexes can also be impacted by function—for example, absence of nasal breathing and occurrence of mouth breathing, leading to a blunting of reflexes and also a progressive absence of responsivity of tongue protruding muscle fibers. It has also been proposed that disruption of sleep by sleep fragmentation can lead to a blunting of many reflexes, including those involved in the stimulation of muscle contraction during inspiration. Additionally, sleep per se has an impact on reflexes such that there is a decrease in reflex activity during non-REM (NREM) sleep, and during REM sleep there is an active inhibition of volitional muscles (and the tongue is a volitional muscle). There are also factors related to gravity: supine or lateral position may have an impact on the collapsibility of UA.

In association with intrinsic factors, there are extrinsic factors that change the size of the UA. Fat deposits that infiltrate the tongue muscles, in particular, and the neck muscles and surrounding soft tissues[1,12] and chronic inflammation that enlarges tissues clearly reduce the UA lumen, as shown by MRI studies in children. Alterations in the anatomic supports of the UA lead to further narrowing of lumen. During the rapid growth period, these factors lead to a vicious cycle, that is, an extrinsic factor reducing the size of UA leads to disturbance of sleep that has an impact on reflexes targeting induction of muscle tension during the vulnerable states of sleep and also leads to a decrease in size of the lumen of the UA, increasing the UA resistance. At a certain point, mouth breathing occurs and another functional change is added that worsens the entire situation. For many years, the physical laws governing airflow in the UA have been studied, with well-known applicationa, such as the Bernoulli principle. Now the fluid-dynamic laws[13] are applied, and these different reflexes, anatomic factors, and functional factors are continuously changing airflow in the lumen, with each component playing a role in the decrease in lumen size and location. Such continuous variability of the points of collapse has been a challenge for appropriate surgical treatments. Nonetheless, the fact remains: the absence of normal stimulation of the orofacial growth centers leads to further abnormal growth.

THE CLINICAL FINDINGS

The understanding of the progressive impact of intrinsic and extrinsic factors in the switch from nasal breathing to mouth breathing and the development of abnormal breathing during sleep have led to a change in the approach to diagnosis and treatment of SDB. Calculation of Pcrit is possible in young children but it is not an easy value to obtain and not enough data are available. On the other hand, clinical evaluation of the oronasal structures can be part of every regular clinical evaluation, starting from birth. For example, at birth, 1 feature that has a long-term impact on

orofacial growth that should be systematically checked, independently of any complaint, is the presence of a short frenulum.[14] Symptoms may be seen early, as in difficulty latching, or later in child development, such as difficulty pronouncing some sounds (variable depending on language), or may just be presence of abnormal orofacial growth picked up by orthodontists or pediatric dentists. Current data show that clipping of the short frenulum should be done during the first month of life, because simple clipping leads to formation of fibrous tissues and persistence of the short frenulum thereafter. Recognition of enlarged adenoids that may, rarely, be present and of an important septum deviation are 2 other early-in-life issues difficult to immediately treat but that need continuous attention and as early treatment as possible. Family history can provide important details on a positive family history of short frenulum but also positive family history of missing 2 or more teeth congenitally. These children should be regularly followed and as early as possible have consideration of radiography to identify presence/absence of permanent teeth roots.

The most important clinical evaluation finding is investigation of the width of the hard palate. It is a difficult measurement to obtain. Normative data indicate that at 40 weeks' gestational age, the width is 20 mm, and during the first year of life there is a clear gain.[15,16] Any impact on orofacial growth stops widening and no change is noted at 6 months and 12 months. Presence of enlarged turbinates can be clearly noted at 6 months and 13 months of age. Tonsils are not enlarged even in premature infants and in toddlers the Friedman scale[17] has been used. Abnormal tonsillar growth seems related to mouth breathing, and enlarged tonsils then accentuate the problem and have a further impact on orofacial growth and mouth breathing.

In the authors' studies, with the exception of the longitudinal study of premature infants, most of the data are obtained on children 2 years and older. At that age, when abnormal orofacial growth or abnormal breathing during sleep is suspected, the Mallampati scale or Mallampati-Friedman scale[18,19] can be obtained as well as the Friedman tonsil scale,[17] width of the hard palate measure at level of lateral incisor, and presence of a short frenulum. Similarly, measurement of the harmonic face (**Fig. 1**) can be obtained,[20] and evaluation of septal deviation and percentage of occupation in nasal cavity by turbinates can be obtained. A dental radiograph and cephalometric evaluation can be obtained as well.

The polysomnogram (PSG) yields a critical piece of information. If apnea and hypopnea are present,

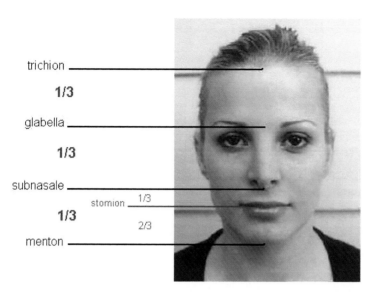

trichion

1/3

glabella

1/3

subnasale

stomion 1/3

1/3

2/3

menton

Fig. 1. Harmonic face. A normal developing face has a normal distribution: measurements of distances from trichion to glabella, from glabella to subnasale, and from subnasale to end of chin should be equal. If 1 segment is longer, there is an abnormal orofacial growth.

there can be little question about the functional consequences of features detected on examination. Still, PSG has issues: it is necessary to recognize electroencephalogram arousal when scoring hypopneas, because oxygen drops are not necessarily common in children with normal cardiopulmonary status and it is also necessary to use the pediatric apnea-hypopnea index (AHI) criteria of less than or equal to 1 event/h as cutoff point.

The PSG can demonstrate much more than the perhaps overly reductionistic AHI (**Fig. 2**), including, most importantly, the presence of flow limitation. This is seen on the nasal cannula flow tracing, although, to be identified, a DC signal must be used, with collection at a sufficient sampling rate and software smoothing filters turned off. The first normative data on flow limitation were obtained in adults by Palombini and colleagues[21] on a representative sample of the general population, and the upper limit of normal cutoff point was 30% of total sleep time. In the authors' study of 500 children 5 years to 13 years old with suspected SDB, the upper limit of normal cutoff point was 20% of sleep time. Flow limitation was defined as follows[22]: (1) flattening of the peak of the nasal cannula pressure transducer wave contour with change in the normal round presentation of the peak of the nasal cannula wave contour during inspiration (**Fig. 3**); (2) at least 4 consecutive breaths must demonstrate the abnormal pattern. The duration of the flow limitation was calculated from the beginning of the inspiratory curve associated with the flattening, until the inspiratory curve returns to a normal round pattern of the curve. For a 30-second epoch, if more than 15 seconds' flow limitation

was observed, the epoch was scored as positive for flow limitation; if there was less than 15 seconds, the epoch was scored as normal breathing.

Another critical item easily identified—if it is looked for—on the PSG is the degree of mouth breathing. Oral breathing can be monitored with a thermistor, without or within an oral scoop. At least 2 different studies looked at normal value for mouth breathing during sleep. Both studies came up with similar results: normal subjects spend approximately 5% of sleep with mouth breathing (range 0%–10% in the authors' study), with an upper limit cutoff point of 15% during sleep identified.[23,24]

These 2 variables are important indicators of abnormal breathing and have been noted in individuals with abnormal hard palate measurement and an AHI maximum at 3 events/h (range 0–3). All abnormal variables were shown to disappear when subjects were placed for 1 months with nasal continuous PAP.

FOLLOW-UP OF INDIVIDUALS AFTER ADENOTONSILLECTOMY

Identification of a breathing abnormality does not always lead to treatment. If enlarged adenoids and/or tonsils were noted, patients frequently accept the treatment recommendation of adenotonsillectomy; however, current data in the literature have indicated that such treatment approach is often not completely successful. A prospective study showed that there is recurrence of abnormal breathing during sleep within 3 years.[25] This systematic study had been preceded by less rigorous studies, indicating that clinical symptoms of SDM recur in early puberty.[26,27]

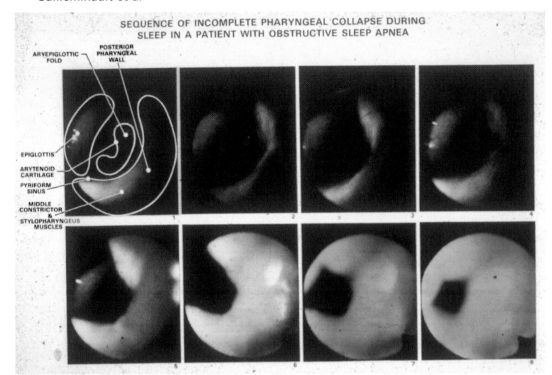

Fig. 2. Video film of UA in sleeping subjects. The films were performed on sleeping subjects during NREM sleep. No local anesthesia was used. Videoscope was placed at same level just after nasal passage: Where does the hypopnea begin? There are 8 different frames from normal opening (frame 1) to important but incomplete collapse (frame 8 [*bottom right*]) Frames 4 to 8 were observed associated with a drop in oxygen saturation of at least 3% at different times in different subjects. But the image obtained showing collapse leading to drop in arterial oxygen saturation (Sao$_2$) of 3% varied. The notion of obstructive hypopnea is vague and variable.

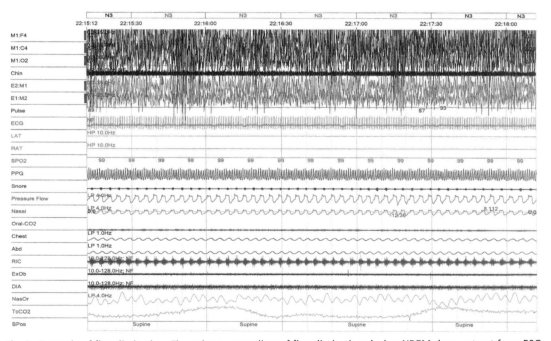

Fig. 3. Example of flow limitation. Five-minute recording of flow limitation during NREM sleep extract from PSG; monitoring with nasal cannula seen on channels 14 and 15—direct recording and modified recording to emphasize flow limitation. The wave contour obtained from the nasal cannula shows a square line and not the round line normally seen during normal breathing. The cutoff top of the wave contour indicates the presence of continuous flow limitation during the selected segment. Note flow limitation here is associated with snoring recorded by neck microphone and presented on channel 19 from top.

OSAS versus UARS: age: 20–39y,40–49y,50–59y,60–69y,>70y.

- Palombini et al-abstract-Sleep-

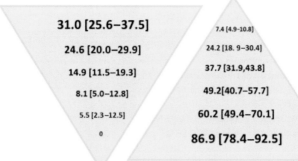

Fig. 4. The opposite triangles from the Brazilian study; 1042 subjects were involved in the study of a representative sample of general population of São Paulo. Individuals with SDB were subdivided in UARS patients and OSA patients, based on PSG findings. In the younger subject groups (18–40 years of age, UARS is prominent while OSAS is rare, in the older age group (over 40 years of age) UARS greatly decreases and OSAS is noted with increased frequency.

PSG confirmation of abnormal AHI, in the presence of abnormal untreated orofacial growth, has been demonstrated. Such abnormal growth was clear in the first study reported, as indicated by cephalometry.[28] Another study performed in the United Kingdom[29] found a frequent recurrence of abnormal AHI in young adulthood. These studies demonstrate that treating children with adenotonsillectomy without checking for and treating abnormal orofacial growth lead to either incomplete resolution or to recurrence of abnormal breathing during sleep as a teenager or young adult.

A more systematic study was performed on children around puberty. At puberty, orofacial growth velocity again increases, with growth involving a counterclockwise rotation of the mandible with vertical increase of the body of the maxilla. If no treatment has been performed before this time to correct abnormal orofacial growth, there are negative consequences on the orofacial development. If the upper teeth do not hit the lower teeth in an appropriate way, a deep overbite occurs, and, later, the upper teeth block the counterclockwise rotation of the mandible; a clockwise rotation occurs, leading to a retroposition of the mandible and further narrowing of the UA. This is only 1 of the possible consequences. With puberty and increased secretion of the sexual hormones, there is enlargement of muscles and soft tissues—more in boys than in girls. This also leads to further narrowing of the UA, with the decrease in size varying

depending of the degree of abnormal orofacial growth and the speed of pubertal changes. As these structural changes occur, a positive feedback loop is reinforced with progressive development of snoring and resultant negative impact on UA reflexes.

The authors, in 1993,[30] reported that young adult subjects presented a symptomatology of UA resistance syndrome (UARS) and since then have progressed to a better understanding of the changes present behind abnormal breathing during sleep. The Brazilian group, in their study of a representative sample of the population of São Paulo,[21] looked at the distribution of abnormal breathing during sleep in those ages 18 years and older. They described "two opposite triangles" (**Fig. 4**), with older adults presenting mostly OSAS and with a large decrease in frequency of UARS.

SUMMARY

Abnormal breathing during sleep began much earlier than recognition of OSA. An understanding of these principles offers an opportunity to recognize and intervene in SDB far earlier in its development, to avoid the many serious and life-altering comorbidities that have been so well associated with OSA. And the only valid treatment goal is restoration of nasal breathing,[31] not only during wakefulness but also during sleep. Absence of normal nasal breathing leads to mouth breathing and development of local inflammation that may become more general progressively, having am impact on on the normal reflexes involved in maintenance of a patent UA. Snoring develops and there are both disuse of normal reflexes and impairment of reflexes caused by both by inflammation and perhaps local vibration[32] related to snoring, the beginning of slow progression toward OSA with comorbidities.

REFERENCES

1. Schwab RJ, Pasirstein M, Pierson R, et al. Identification of upper airway anatomic risk factors for obstructive sleep apnea with volumetric magnetic resonance imaging. Am J Respir Crit Care Med 2003;168(5):522–30.
2. Guilleminault C, Eldridge F, Simmons F, et al. Sleep apnea in eight children. Pediatrics 1976;58:23–30.
3. Redline S, Tishler PV, Tosteson TD, et al. The familial aggregation of obstructive sleep apnea. Am J Respir Crit Care Med 1995;151:682–7.
4. Guilleminault C, Partinen M, Hollman K, et al. Familial aggregates in obstructive sleep apnea syndrome. Chest 1995;107:1545–51.
5. Mathur R, Douglas NJ. Family studies in patients with the sleep apnea-hypopnea syndrome. Ann Intern Med 1995;122:174–8.
6. Guilleminault C, Huang Y-S. From oral facial dysfunction to dysmorphism and the onset of pediatric OSA. Sleep Med Rev 2018;40:203–14.
7. Couly G, Levaillant JM, Bault JP, et al. Oralit_du fetus. France: Sauramps medical montpellier; 2015. p. 1–138.
8. Levaillant JM, Bault JP, Benoit B, et al. La face foetale normale et pathologique, aspects_echographiques. France: Sauramps Medical Montpellier; 2013. p. 1–120.
9. Aknin JJ, editor. La croissance cranio-faciale. Paris: SID Publ; 2007. p. 1–254.
10. Guilleminault C, Akhtar F. Pediatrics sleep-disordered-breathing: new evidences on its development. Sleep Med Rev 2015;14:1–11.
11. Huang YS, Paiva T, Hsu JF, et al. Sleep and breathing in premature infants at 6 months of age. BMC Pediatrics 2014;14:303.
12. Arens R, McDonough JM, Corbin AM, et al. Upper airway size analysis by magnetic resonance imaging of children with obstructive sleep apnea syndrome. Am J Respir Crit Care Med 2003;167:65–70.
13. Powell NB, Mihaescu M, Mylavarapu G, et al. Patterns in pharyngeal airflow associated with sleep-disordered breathing. Sleep Med 2011;12:966–74.
14. Guilleminault C, Huseni S, Lo L. A frequent phenotype for paediatrics obstructive sleep apnea: short lingual frenulum. ERJ Open Res 2016;2:00043–7.
15. Page DC. "Real" early orthodontic treatment. From birth to age 8. Funct Orthod 2003;20(1–2):48–54, 56-58.
16. Bahr D. Nobody ever told me that Arlington Tx sensory development. 2010. p. 9.
17. Friedman M, Tanyeri H, La Rosa M, et al. Clinical predictors of obstructive sleep apnea. Laryngoscope 1999;109:1901–7.
18. Mallampati SR, Gatt SP, Gugino LD, et al. A clinical sign to predict difficult tracheal intubation: a prospective study. Can Anaesth Soc J 1985;32:429–34.
19. Friedman M, Ibrahim H, Bass L. Clinical staging for sleep-disordered breathing. Otolaryngol Head Neck Surg 2002;127:13–21.
20. Kim JH, Guilleminault C. The naso-maxillary complex, the mandible and sleep disordered-breathing. Sleep Breath 2011;15:185–93.
21. Palombini LO, Tufik S, Rapoport DM, et al. Inspiratory flow limitation in a normal population of adults in Sao Paulo, Brazil. Sleep 2013;36:1663–8.
22. Arora N, Meskill G, Guilleminault C. The role of flow limitation as an important diagnostic tool and clinical finding in mild sleep-disordered breathing. Sleep Sci 2015;8(3):134–42.
23. Fitzpatrick MF, McLean H, Urton AM, et al. Effect of nasal or oral breathing route on upper airway resistance during sleep. Eur Respir J 2003;22(5):827–32.
24. Lee S-Y, Guilleminault C, Chiu H-Y, et al. Mouth breathing, "nasal disuse," and pediatric sleep-disordered breathing. Sleep and Breathing 2015; 19(4):1257–64.
25. Huang YS, Guilleminault C, Lee LA, et al. Treatment outcomes of adenotonsillectomy for children with obstructive sleep apnea: a prospective longitudinal study. Sleep 2014;37:71–80.
26. Guilleminault C, Huang YS, Quo S, et al. Teenage sleep disordered breathing: recurrence of syndrome. Sleep Med 2013;14:37–44.
27. Guilleminault C, Huang YS, Monteyrol PJ, et al. Critical role of myofacial reeducation in sleep-disordered breathing. Sleep Med 2013;14:518–25.
28. Guilleminault C, Partinen M, Praud JP, et al. Morphometric facial changes and obstructive sleep apnea in adolescent. J Peds 1989;114:997–9.
29. Tasker C, Crosby JH, Stradling JR. Evidence for persistence of upper airway narrowing during sleep, 12 years after adenotonsillectomy. Arch Dis Child 2002;86:34–7.
30. Guilleminault C, Stoohs R, Clerk A, et al. A cause of excessive daytime sleepiness. The upper airway resistance syndrome. Chest 1993;104:781–7.
31. Guilleminault C, Sullivan SS. Toward restauration of continuous nasal breathing as the ultimate treatment goal in pediatric obstructive sleep apnea Enliven. Pediatr Neonatol Biol 2014;1:1–7.
32. Friberg D, Ansved T, Borg K, et al. Histological indications of a progressive snorers disease in an upper-airway muscle. Am J Resp Crit Care Med 1998;157:586–93.

Anatomic and Pathophysiologic Considerations in Surgical Treatment of Obstructive Sleep Apnea

Srinivas Kishore Sistla, MBBS, MS (ENT)[a],*,
Vijaya Krishnan Paramasivan, MBBS, DNB, DLO[b],
Vikas Agrawal, MBBS, MS (ENT)[c,1]

KEYWORDS

- OSAS • Anatomy of upper airway • Pathophysiology of OSAS
- Skeletal framework of upper airway in OSAS • Genetics in OSAS • Loop gain • Pcrit
- Starling resistor

KEY POINTS

- Evaluation of the upper airway is key for a successful surgical management. Proper evaluation can be done only with a good understanding of the anatomy and pathophysiology of the upper airway.
- Retrognathia, adenotonsillar hypertrophy, enlarged tongue, lateral pharyngeal wall thickening, and parapharyngeal fat pads are important anatomic risk factors.
- Upper airway collapsibility and arousal response are heightened in apneic patients.
- Elevated loop gain leads to an overshoot of ventilator response in obstructive sleep apnea (OSA), contributing to ventilator instability.
- The understanding of pathophysiology of OSAS is evolving, because all the anatomic and physiologic characteristics discussed have genetic predisposition. Gene therapy may play a pivotal role in the future.

INTRODUCTION

Obstructive sleep apnea (OSA) is a condition characterized by recurrent episodes of restricted airflow secondary to obstruction of the upper airways during sleep.

From a purely anatomic perspective, a narrow upper airway is generally more prone to collapse than a larger one. Accordingly, on the whole, the cross-sectional area of the upper airway as measured by imaging during wakefulness is reduced in patients with OSA compared with subjects without OSA.[1] Furthermore, the arrangement of the surrounding soft tissues appears to be altered in patients with OSA, which may place the upper airway at risk for collapse.[1]

Disclosure statement: No Disclosure.
[a] Department of ENT, Star Hospital, Block B, Road Number 10, Banjara Hills, Hyderabad 500034, Telangana, India; [b] Department of Snoring & Sleep Disorders, Madras ENT Research Foundation, 1, Ist Cross Street, Off II Main Road, Raja Annamalaipuram, Chennai 600028, Tamil Nadu, India; [c] Department of ENT, Specialty ENT Hospital, Kandivali East, Mumbai 400101, Maharashtra, India
[1] Present address: Madras ENT Research Foundation, 1, Ist Cross Street, Off II Main Road, Raja Annamalaipuram, Chennai 600028.
* Corresponding author.
E-mail address: drsrinivas.sistla@gmail.com

Sleep Med Clin 14 (2019) 21–31
https://doi.org/10.1016/j.jsmc.2018.11.003
1556-407X/19/© 2018 Elsevier Inc. All rights reserved.

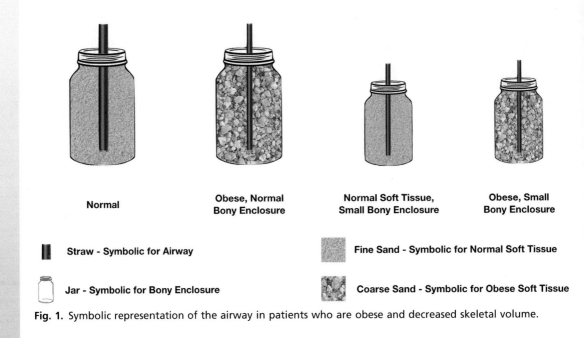

Fig. 1. Symbolic representation of the airway in patients who are obese and decreased skeletal volume.

One of the major tenets of upper airway surgery is to understand the concept of skeletal frame work and the soft tissue within (**Fig. 1**).

SOFT TISSUE

The soft tissue component of the upper airway is divided into 3 sections: the nasopharynx, oropharynx, and hypopharynx (**Fig. 2**).

ROLE OF NOSE AND NASOPHARYNX

Humans naturally breathe through the nose, particularly during sleep, when the daily oral fraction of breathing, estimated at 7%, drops to 4% during sleep.[2] Although during wakefulness both nasal and oral resistances are equal, nasal resistance is lower than the oral at night, but increases in supine position. Nasal obstruction can occur secondary to alar collapse, deviated septum, turbinate hypertrophy, rhinosinusitis, polyps, nonallergic rhinitis, septal tubercles, and concha bullosa (**Fig. 3**).

Nasal congestion has been associated with a 3-fold increase in the incidence of snoring and daytime sleepiness. The nasopharynx extends from the posterior margin of the nasal turbinates; it sits above the soft palate and continues inferiorly with the oropharynx. The roof and posterior wall are occupied by adenoids (**Fig. 4**), which when inflamed can partially obstruct the upper airway. The adenoids and tonsillar hypertrophy (**Figs. 5** and **6**), when accompanied by allergic rhinitis, can result in mild to moderate OSA in children. Studies indicate that acute nasal obstruction could increase the Apnea-Hypopnea Index, prolong rapid eye movement (REM) latency, and increase non-REM (NREM) sleep. However, just treating the nose in isolation seldom cures the disease.

OROPHARYNX

The hard and soft palate form the roof of the oral cavity, and the tongue forms the floor. The

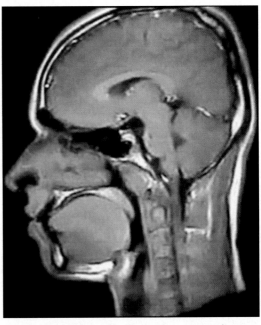

Fig. 2. Midsagittal MRI illustrating anatomic structures of interest.

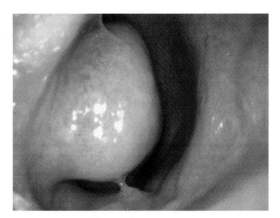

Fig. 3. Hypertrophied inferior turbinate.

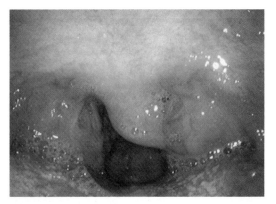

Fig. 5. Hypertrophied tonsils on oral cavity examination.

oropharynx within the upper airway extends from the posterior end of hard palate to the upper surface of the hyoid and is of importance due to its propensity to collapse. The anterior part of oropharynx is formed by the posterior part of the tongue and the soft palate, whereas the posterior part is formed by the pharyngeal constrictor muscles. The lateral pharyngeal walls are formed by the pharyngeal constrictors, muscles of the extrinsic tongue, muscles of the soft palate, and the larynx. Other structures that contribute to upper airway lumen, located in the retropalatal area, are the palatine tonsils and parapharyngeal fat pads.

SURGICAL LANDMARKS OF SOFT PALATE
Palatal Dimple

If the oral surface of the palate is observed while a subject says "Ah," the palate is seen to arch, and convexities occur at the point, or points, of maximum excursion. The apices of these concavities can be termed palatal "dimples" usually at the

junction of the middle and posterior thirds of the soft palate. The measurements of dimple position (mean 24 mm from the hard palate in an average palate of length 40 mm). The relationship of dimples to levator muscles is that they occurred at the point where levator and palatopharyngeus muscles intermingle, close to the posterior limit of the levator.[3]

Posterior Nasal Spine

The medial end of the posterior border of the horizontal plate of palatine bone is the posterior nasal spine for the attachment of the musculus uvulae.

Pterygomandibular Raphe

Pterygomandibular raphe is a ligamentous band of the buccopharyngeal fascia, attached superiorly to the pterygoid hamulus of the medial pterygoid plate, and inferiorly to the posterior end of the mylohyoid line of the mandible.

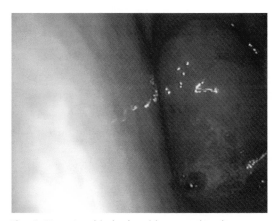

Fig. 4. Hypertrophied adenoid on nasal endoscopy.

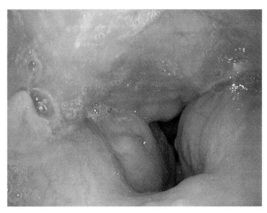

Fig. 6. Hypertrophied tonsils, view from the nasopharynx.

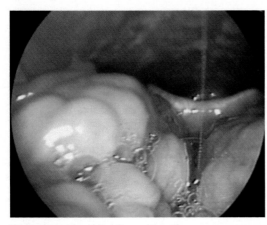

Fig. 7. Hypertrophied lingual tonsils.

Pterygoid Hamulus

Pterygoid hamulus is a hooklike process at the lower extremity of the medial pterygoid plate of the sphenoid bone. Around this, the tendon of the tensor veli palatini glides.

HYPOPHARYNX

The tongue has both extrinsic and intrinsic muscle groups. The oropharyngeal surface may be filled with lingual tonsils, often secondary to reflux and postnasal drip (**Fig. 7**).

The 4 extrinsic tongue muscles are the genioglossus, hyoglossus, palatoglossus, and styloglossus. The genioglossus is the largest pharyngeal dilator muscle. All of these muscles are innervated by the hypoglossal nerve except the palatoglossus, which is innervated by the pharyngeal plexus (**Fig. 8**). The intrinsic muscles are confined to the tongue. The size of the tongue is an important risk factor for OSA.

The hypoglossal nerve is a critical component in the motor control of upper airway dilatation. The muscle fibers in the posterior part of the tongue are fatigue resistant, thereby sustaining the forward tongue position and preventing its collapse into the retroglossal area. This mechanism is the basis for the proximal hypoglossal nerve stimulation, which can be used to treat OSA.[4] An important surgical anatomic landmark in performing tongue base surgery is the lingual hypoglossal bundle.

LANDMARKS FOR THE LINGUAL ARTERY IN RELATION TO THE FORAMEN CECUM

- 2.7 cm inferior and 1.6 cm lateral to the foramen cecum (FC) (**Fig. 9**)

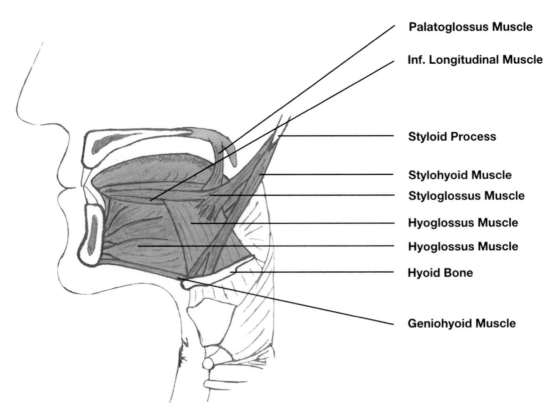

Palatoglossus Muscle

Inf. Longitudinal Muscle

Styloid Process

Stylohyoid Muscle

Styloglossus Muscle

Hyoglossus Muscle

Hyoglossus Muscle

Hyoid Bone

Geniohyoid Muscle

Fig. 8. Intrinsic and extrinsic muscles of the tongue.

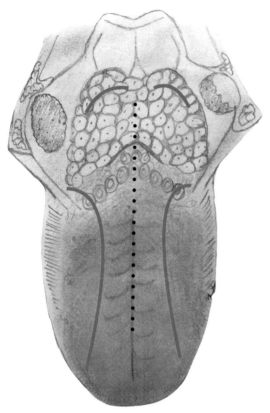

Fig. 9. Course of the lingual artery.

- 2.77 cm inferior and 1.1 cm medial to the lateral tongue margin at the level of the FC
- Within 1.5 cm superior to the hyoid bone (mean 0.9 cm)

The lateral wall of the pharynx plays an important role in the pathogenesis of OSA. A recent study evaluating the role of parapharyngeal fat in the predisposition to OSA used MRI to examine pharyngeal anatomy. Patients with retropalatal airway closure had a higher percentage of parapharyngeal and soft palate fat, whereas patients with retroglossal airway closure had an increased volume of the tongue and parapharyngeal fat pad (**Fig. 10**).

The structures in the hypopharynx, such as the lingual tonsils, can have a potential role in OSA.[5] Epiglottic prolapse during inspiration has been described, which accounts for 13%. A suprahyoid epiglottidectomy is reported as a curative procedure (**Fig. 11**).[6]

SKELETAL FRAME WORK OF UPPER AIRWAY

Maxillomandibular advancement is the most complex upper airway surgery, but excluding tracheostomy, this procedure has the best record of success as a treatment of OSA. The maxilla and the mandible are advanced together, and both upper and lower teeth are moved to maintain adequate occlusion (**Fig. 12**).

Therefore, it is very important to perceive the principle and the contribution of skeletal framework, which encloses the collapsible upper airway to understand the pathophysiology of OSAS.

SKELETAL CLASSIFICATION OF MAXILLARY MANDIBULAR COMPLEX

It is important to understand the relationship between the maxilla and the mandible, in an anteroposterior direction:

Class I: The maxilla and the mandible are in harmony with each other.

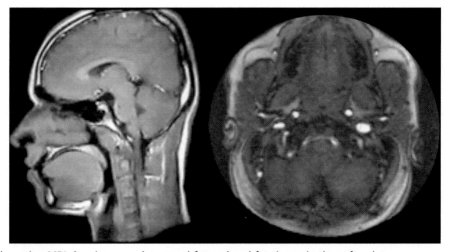

Fig. 10. Sleep cine MRI showing parapharyngeal fat pad and fat tissues in the soft palate.

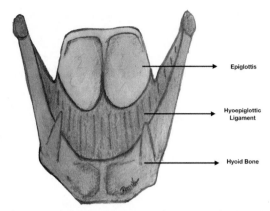

Fig. 11. Epiglottis with its attachment to the hyoid through the hyoepiglottic ligament.

Class II: The maxilla lies ahead of the mandible with reference to anterior cranial base; in other words, the mandible is retrognathic.

Class III: The maxilla lies posterior to the mandible with reference to anterior cranial base; in other words, the mandible is prognathic.

The anterior cranial base relates to the position of the maxilla, whereas the posterior cranial base relates to the positions of the glenoid fossa and the mandible.

For male patients with OSA, at the age of 4 years, the angle decreases from 132.2° ± 5.9° to 129.4°± 5.4° at the age of 20 years, and in female patients

with OSA, it decreases from 132.9°± 4.9° to 131.7°± 4.2° at the age of 20 years.

INCREASE IN CRANIAL BASE LENGTH

It is important to understand the influence of cranial base length on the relationship between maxilla and mandible; with an increase in cranial base length, there is a tendency toward skeletal II pattern (retrognathic) (**Fig. 13**).

DECREASE IN CRANIAL BASE ANGLE

With an increase in cranial base angle, there is a tendency toward skeletal II pattern. When the angle reduces, the skeletal pattern is likely to tend toward a class III (prognathic) relationship (**Fig. 14**).

Most studies show that individuals with larger cranial base angles and or larger anterior and posterior cranial base lengths tend to be retrognathic (ie, class II), whereas those with smaller lengths and angles tend to be prognathic (ie, class III).[7]

CLASSIFICATION OF SOFT PALATE

Soft palate is classified based on the angle it makes with the hard palate. The more acute the angle of the soft palate in relation to the hard palate, more muscular activity will be necessary to effect velopharyngeal closure (closing of the nasopharynx) (**Fig. 15**).

HOUSE CLASSIFICATION OF PALATAL THROAT FORM

Class I is large and normal in form with a relatively immovable band of resilient tissue 5 to 12 mm distal to a line drawn across distal edge of the tuberosities with an acute angle of 10°.[8]

Class II is medium size and normal in form with a relatively immovable resilient band of tissue 3 to 5 mm distal to a line drawn across distal edge of the tuberosities with an angle of 45°.

Class III usually accompanies a small maxilla. The curtain of soft tissues turns down abruptly 3 to 5 mm anterior to a line drawn across distal edge of the tuberosities with an angle of 70°.

PATHOPHYSIOLOGIC CONSIDERATION

Considerable heterogeneity exists in the mechanism of OSA in patients.[9] The complex interaction among pharyngeal dilator tone, arousal threshold, respiratory control instability, and changes in lung volume during sleep play an important role in OSA.

The factors that govern the pathophysiology are as follows.

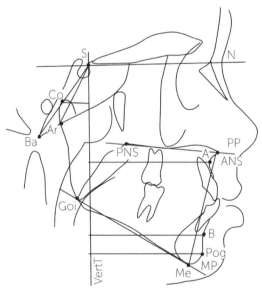

S - N : Anterior cranial base

S - Ar, S - Ba : Posterior cranial base

Fig. 12. Cephalometric analysis of anterior and posterior cranial base.

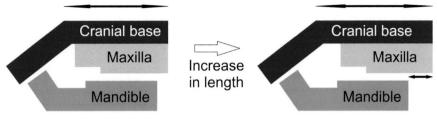

Fig. 13. Increase in cranial base length showing class II pattern.

Upper Airway Collapsibility

Upper airway collapsibility occurs due to the variation in transmural pressure and the decrease in the longitudinal tension of the pharynx. MRI studies done on OSA patients indicate that the airway is anteroposteriorly elliptical because of the thicker lateral pharyngeal walls influenced by the parapharyngeal fat pads.

The pressure required to maintain patency of the upper airway is called the pharyngeal closing pressure (P_{crit}). P_{crit} has been shown to correlate with OSA severity.[10] When the principles of a Starling resistor are applied, the pharyngeal airway can be conceptualized as a collapsible tube surrounded by tissue within a bony box (**Fig. 16**).

The luminal size is determined by the properties of the tube and the transmural pressure, which is the difference between pressures inside and outside the tube. An increase in the outside tissue pressure will promote luminal narrowing.

P_{crit} will increase as tissue pressure increases, which could occur from a reduction in size of the bony box, for example, micrognathia, midthird hypoplasia of the face, or by adenotonsillar hypertrophy, macroglossia, or obesity. Weight loss has been shown to reduce P_{crit},[11] and the resolution of sleep-disordered breathing depends on the degree of P_{crit} reduction.

Similarly, a stepwise advancement of the mandible in apneic patients leads to dose-dependent reductions in P_{crit}.[12]

Upper Airway Dilator Activity

In OSA patients, it has been found that the upper airway dilator tone is higher than normal in subjects during wakefulness, and this maintains an open airway. During sleep, this tone decreases, thereby leading to airway instability.

Local reflexes generated by negative pharyngeal pressure during sleep modulate an increase in both genioglossus and tensor palatine tone, especially in the supine position.

Upper airway dilator muscle activity and recruitability are considerably studied in OSAS patients. High-frequency sampling techniques have recently been used to define single motor units (SMUs) within the genioglossus. These SMU techniques allow sorting of individual motor units within the genioglossus muscle, which has shown considerable complexity. These SMU techniques when applied to the genioglossus electromyograph allow insights into cellular activity within the hypoglossal motor nucleus, offering the possibility of novel therapeutic targets for some OSA patients. During stable sleep in healthy individuals, genioglossal activity is maintained at or above waking levels.

Genioglossus is more active in apnea patients during wakefulness, and at sleep onset, this activity falls to a greater extent. During stable NREM sleep, the combination of mechanical and chemical stimuli is much more effective at increasing upper airway muscle activity than either stimulus alone.

Lung Volumes

Caudal traction and elongation of the airway reduce P_{crit} through stiffening the airway and mitigating the surrounding tissue pressures.

The supine position reduces lung volumes in apneic patients, which decreases caudal traction on the airway. An increase in end-expiratory lung

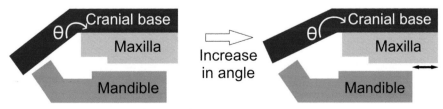

Fig. 14. Increase in cranial base angle showing class III pattern.

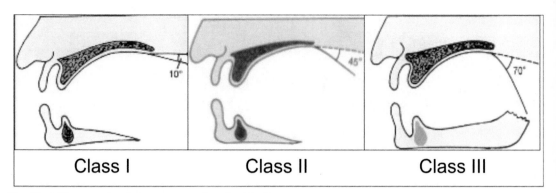

Fig. 15. Different palatal phenotype as described by House.

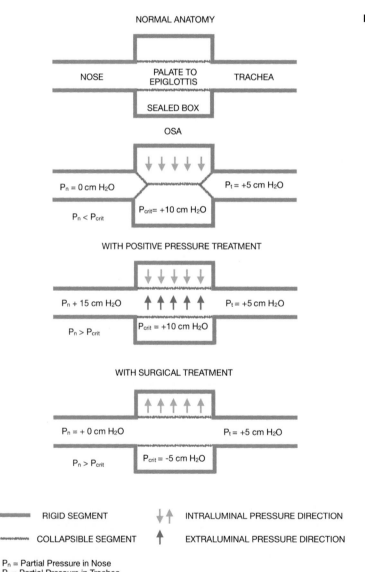

Fig. 16. Starling resistor model.

P_n = Partial Pressure in Nose
P_t = Partial Pressure in Trachea
P_{crit} = Partial Pressure required to keep trachea open (Critical Partial Pressure)
All pressure values are arbitrary, just to make it easy to understand.

volume using continuous positive airway pressure (CPAP) has been shown to substantially reduce apnea severity and improve sleep architecture.[13]

Arousal Thresholds

Apneas are usually followed by arousals, which are thought to be mediated via negative intrathoracic pressure generation; however, it can be terminated without an arousal by the stimuli coming from the chemoreceptors and intrapharyngeal pressure receptors.[14]

OSA impairs the arousal threshold, and therefore, apneic patients need greater inspiratory efforts to trigger an arousal.[15] This means that apneic patients experience prolonged event duration because of the heightened length of inspiratory effort required to trigger an arousal. On the contrary, a low arousal threshold can impact the sleep architecture, resulting in excessive daytime sleepiness.

Ventilatory Control

The respiratory response to airway collapsibility and arousal can be conceptualized as "loop gain," which refers to the response of the respiratory center relative to the intensity of the input.[16]

A high loop gain is an unstable, robust ventilatory response to a stimulus, and lower loop gain is a poor response to a similar stimulus.

In a study, Edwards and colleagues[17] showed that acetazolamide reduced the ventilator response

to spontaneous arousal in patients with OSA treated with CPAP and improved ventilatory instability.

Surface Tension

Patients with OSA appear to have increased surface forces acting on the upper airway. Nasal breathing may reduce, and oral breathing may increase, surface tension forces. Thus, changes in breathing route in OSA may be one of many factors contributing to the elevated levels of surface tension observed in OSA.[18]

Pharyngeal Neuropathy

Inflammation and denervation affect the oral mucosa and upper airway muscles in patients with OSA. This results in selective impairment in the ability to detect mechanical stimuli in the upper airway of patients with OSA and snorers (**Fig. 17**).

IMPACT OF RISK FACTORS
Obesity

Obese patients with OSA have increased fat deposits in the soft tissue surrounding the upper airway, including in the soft palate.[19] This finding of a small increase in upper airway soft tissue volume in apneic patients compared with normal controls was confirmed in Japanese patients.[20] Furthermore, a small decrease of 17 cm^3 in upper airway volume from overall weight loss (average of 7.8 kg) led to a 31% decrease in the apnea-hypopnea index.[21] A reduction in

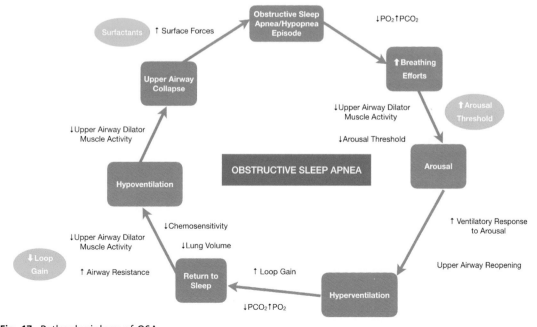

Fig. 17. Pathophysiology of OSA.

functional residual capacity (FRC) is seen in obese individuals, and decreased upper airway patency from low FRC is an additional mechanism contributing to OSA in obese patients; hence, weight loss and increase in FRC improve airway patency.

Male Sex

An increase in pharyngeal airway length and soft palate area may explain the higher predisposition to pharyngeal collapsibility in men.[22] Arousals from sleep in men are associated with a greater ventilatory response and with hypoventilation on falling back asleep compared with women, worsening in the supine position.

Age

The prevalence of OSA increases with age, which plateaus after 65 years of age.[23] Increased parapharyngeal fat and upper airway narrowing have been observed in elderly patients.[24] Studies indicate that patients have an increased vulnerability from longer airways with age.[25]

Genetics

There is a clear familial basis to the development of OSA irrespective of obesity.[26] Fifty studies using linkage analysis have provided initial insight into the potential link between specific areas of the genome and OSA pathogenesis.[27] Anatomy (obesity, craniofacial structure) clearly have genetic basis. Traits, such as the size of the upper airway soft tissue structures, ventilatory control abnormalities, and respiratory responses to apnea during sleep, may also have a genetic basis.[28,29]

SUMMARY

Evaluation of the upper airway is key for a successful surgical management. Proper evaluation can be done only with a good understanding of the anatomy and pathophysiology of the upper airway. Retrognathia, adenotonsillar hypertrophy, enlarged tongue, lateral pharyngeal wall thickening, and parapharyngeal fat pads are important anatomic risk factors. The understanding of pathophysiology of OSA is evolving. Upper airway collapsibility and arousal response are heightened in apneic patients. Elevated loop gain leads to an overshoot of ventilator response in OSA, contributing to ventilator instability. Because all the anatomic and physiologic characteristics discussed have genetic predisposition, gene therapy may play a pivotal role in the future.

REFERENCES

1. Schwab RJ, Gupta KB, Gefter WB, et al. Upper airway and soft tissue anatomy in normal subjects and patients with sleep-disordered breathing: significance of the lateral pharyngeal walls. Am J Respir Crit Care Med 1995;152:1673–89.
2. Fitzpatrick MF, Driver HS, Chatha N, et al. Partitioning of inhaled ventilation between the nasal and oral routes during sleep in normal subjects. J Appl Physiol 2003;94(3):883–90.
3. Boorman G, Sommerlad BC. Levator palati and palatal dimples: their anatomy, relationship and clinical significance. Br J Plast Surg 1985;38: 326–38.
4. Zaidi FN, Meadows P, Jacobowitz O, et al. Tongue anatomy and physiology, the scientific basis for a novel targeted neurostimulation system designed for the treatment of obstructive sleep apnea. Neuromodulation 2012. https://doi.org/10.1111/j. 1525-1403.2012.00514.x.
5. Suzuki K, Kawakatsu K, Hattori C, et al. Application of lingual tonsillectomy to sleep apnea syndrome involving lingual tonsils. Acta Otolaryngol Suppl 2003;550:65–71.
6. Catalfumo FJ, Golz A, Westerman ST, et al. The epiglottis and obstructive sleep apnoea syndrome. J Laryngol Otol 1998;112(10):940–3.
7. Björk A. Cranial base development. Am J Orthod 1955;41(3):198–225.
8. House MM. The relationship of oral examination to dental diagnosis. J Prosthet Dent 1958;8(2):208–19.
9. Eckert DJ, Malhotra A. Pathophysiology of adult obstructive sleep apnea. Proc Am Thorac Soc 2008;5:144–53.
10. Issa FG, Sullivan CE. Upper airway closing pressures in obstructive sleep apnea. J Appl Physiol 1984;57:520–7.
11. Schwartz AR, Gold AR, Schubert N, et al. Effect of weight loss on upper airway collapsibility in obstructive sleep apnea. Am Rev Respir Dis 1991;144: 494–8.
12. Kato J, Isono S, Tanaka A, et al. Dose-dependent effects of mandibular advancement on pharyngeal mechanics and nocturnal oxygenation in patients with sleep-disordered breathing. Chest 2000;117: 1065–72.
13. Heinzer RC, Stanchina ML, Malhotra A, et al. Effect of increased lung volume on sleep disordered breathing in patients with sleep apnoea. Thorax 2006;61:435–9.
14. Younes M. Role of arousals in the pathogenesis of obstructive sleep apnea. Am J Respir Crit Care Med 2004;169:623–33.
15. Berry RB, Kouchi KG, Der DE, et al. Sleep apnea impairs the arousal response to airway occlusion. Chest 1996;109:1490–6.

16. Khoo MC, Kronauer RE, Strohl KP, et al. Factors inducing periodic breathing in humans: a general model. J Appl Physiol 1982;53:644–59.

17. Malhotra A, Jordan AS. Did fat boy Joe need hormone replacement? Sleep 2006;29:16–8.

18. Verma M, Seto-Poon M, Wheatley JR, et al. Influence of breathing route on upper airway lining liquid surface tension in humans. J Physiol 2006;574:859–66.

19. Shelton KE, Woodson H, Gay S, et al. Pharyngeal fat in obstructive sleep apnea. Am Rev Respir Dis 1993; 148:462–6.

20. Eckert DJ, Saboisky JP, Jordan AS, et al. A secondary reflex suppression phase is present in genioglossus but not tensor palatini in response to negative upper airway pressure. J Appl Physiol 2010;108(6):1619–24.

21. Gleeson K, Zwillich CW, White DP. The influence of increasing ventilatory effort on arousal from sleep. Am Rev Respir Dis 1990;142:295–300.

22. Malhotra A, Huang Y, Fogel RB, et al. The male predisposition to pharyngeal collapse: importance of airway length. Am J Respir Crit Care Med 2002; 166:1388–95.

23. Bixler EO, Vgontzas AN, Ten Have T, et al. Effects of age on sleep apnea in men: I, prevalence and severity. Am J Respir Crit Care Med 1998;157: 144–8.

24. Malhotra A, Huang Y, Fogel R, et al. Aging influences on pharyngeal anatomy and physiology: the predisposition to pharyngeal collapse. Am J Med 2006;119:72.e9-14.

25. Edwards BA, O'Driscoll DM, Ali A, et al. Aging and sleep: physiology and pathophysiology. Semin Respir Crit Care Med 2010;31(5):618–33.

26. Strohl KP, Saunders NA, Feldman NT, et al. Obstructive sleep apnea in family members. N Engl J Med 1978;299:969–73.

27. Mathur R, Douglas NJ. Family studies in patients with the sleep apnea–hypopnea syndrome. Ann Intern Med 1995;122:174–8.

28. Larkin EK, Patel SR, Redline S, et al. Apolipoprotein E and obstructive sleep apnea: evaluating whether a candidate gene explains a linkage peak. Genet Epidemiol 2006;30:101–10.

29. Redline S, Leitner J, Arnold J, et al. Ventilatory control abnormalities in familial sleep apnea. Am J Respir Crit Care Med 1997;156:155–60.

Drug-Induced Sleep Endoscopy in Treatment Options Selection

Khai Beng Chong, MBBS[a],*, Andrea De Vito, MD, PhD[b],
Claudio Vicini, MD[b]

KEYWORDS

- Obstructive sleep apnea • Sleep endoscopy • Sedation endoscopy • Upper airway
- Treatment selection

KEY POINTS

- Drug-induced sleep endoscopy is a safe and practical technique to evaluate the dynamic upper airway collapse during sleep.
- There is still a lack of consensus on the sedation drugs and technique, monitoring of sedation depth, and classification of upper airway collapse for drug-induced sleep endoscopy.
- Drug-induced sleep endoscopy is useful to improve treatment options selection for patients with obstructive sleep apnea, especially for those who are unable to accept or tolerate continuous positive airway pressure therapy.

INTRODUCTION

Endoscopic evaluation of the upper airway is an important part of the comprehensive assessment of patients with obstructive sleep apnea (OSA). The aim of this review is to help guide the treatment modality tailored for each individual patient, especially for those who cannot tolerate continuous positive airway pressure therapy.

Awake upper airway endoscopy can be done safely in the office setting for patients with OSA. Awake assessment is useful to evaluate any anatomic variant of the upper airway structures such as deviated nasal septum, turbinates hypertrophy, and adenotonsillar hypertrophy and to rule out pathologic obstruction such as nasal polyps and tumors. However, awake upper airway assessment is less useful to predict the dynamic upper airway soft tissue collapse that occurs

during sleep.[1] The Friedman staging system is a widely used awake anatomic assessment of the palatine tonsil size, tongue position, lingual tonsil hypertrophy, and body mass index to identify potential surgical candidates.[2] Although it does not replace assessment of airway during sleep, the Friedman staging system is useful to help identify patients who do not need further sleep endoscopy assessment.[2]

Borowiecki and colleagues[3] were the first to publish a study on endoscopic upper airway assessment in natural sleep for subjects with OSA. The study was published in 1978 describing the early understanding of the upper airway collapse in OSA when it was still a poorly understood newly termed medical condition.[3] Although it was a promising evaluation tool, it was not done outside research settings because it was uncomfortable and not practical to perform

Disclosure Statement: Nil.
^a Department of Otorhinolaryngology, Tan Tock Seng Hospital, 11 Jalan Tan Tock Seng, Singapore 308433, Singapore; ^b Head and Neck Department, ENT and Oral Surgery Unit, Morgagni-Pierantoni Hospital, AUSL of Romagna, Via Carlo Forlanini 34, Forlì 47121, Italy
* Corresponding author.
E-mail addresses: khai_beng_chong@ttsh.com.sg; ckhaibeng@hotmail.com

Sleep Med Clin 14 (2019) 33–40
https://doi.org/10.1016/j.jsmc.2018.11.001
1556-407X/19/© 2018 Elsevier Inc. All rights reserved.

endoscopy for each patient over a few hours at night in natural sleep.

In 1991, Croft and Pringle[4] were the first to describe upper airway endoscopy under bolus midazolam sedation. They named the new assessment technique sleep nasendoscopy.[4] Croft and Pringle[4] described direct visualization of different levels of obstruction that may be useful in choosing surgical treatment options. Since then, sedation endoscopy of the upper airway has evolved in technique and gained significant popularity with an almost exponential increase in the number of articles published in literature.[5] Many terminologies were used including sleep nasendoscopy, sleep endoscopy, drug-induced sleep endoscopy (DISE), fiberoptic sleep endoscopy and drug-induced sedation endoscopy.[5] For our review, the terminology used will be drug-induced sleep endoscopy (DISE).

DISE is a practical compromise compared with natural sleep endoscopy for the assessment of the dynamic upper airway collapse during sleep. We review DISE in adults, including its indications, technique, evaluation of upper airway collapse, and application for treatment options selection. We are not discussing pediatric DISE because its use in children is still not well-established with few published reports in the literature.[6]

INDICATIONS

The aim of DISE is to identify the site and pattern of upper airway obstruction to help guide treatment selection for the following groups:

1. Patients with OSA who are unable to accept or tolerate continuous positive airway pressure.[7]
2. Patients with socially problematic primary snoring.[5]
3. Patients who failed previous upper airway surgery for OSA.[8]
4. Patients considering non–continuous positive airway pressure treatment options for OSA such as surgery, a mandibular advancement device (MAD), positional therapy, or combination therapy.[9]

CONTRAINDICATIONS

DISE should be avoided if the risk of the procedure is unacceptably high for the following groups:

1. Patients with significant medical risk, with American Society of Anesthesiologists physical status class IV or worse.[5]
2. Pregnant patients.[5]
3. Patients with known allergy to DISE drugs.[5]

DISE is relatively contraindicated for the following groups:

1. Patients with morbid obesity.[5]
2. Patients with markedly severe OSA (an apnea–hypopnea index of >70 per hour).[9]

TECHNIQUE
Settings

DISE can be safely done in the operating theater, endoscopy suite, or office setting. Patients are fasted before DISE to minimize the risk of aspiration during the procedure. Comfortable room temperature with dim lights and a quiet environment will simulate natural sleep condition. The team performing the DISE usually consists of 1 endoscopist, 1 anesthetist (or anesthesia-trained individual), and an assistant (usually a nurse).

Equipment

Basic anesthesia monitoring, such as oxygen saturation, cardiac monitoring, and blood pressure, is used for the procedure. Instruments for drug delivery such as infusion pump or target-controlled infusion should be ready before the procedure. Supplemental oxygen via nasal cannula, face mask, or bag and mask are usually not used, but should be available if necessary. A resuscitation trolley should be nearby in case of emergency. A thin flexible endoscope, ideally with video recording, is used for the airway assessment. The ability to record the snoring intensity will be good, although nonessential.

Monitoring of Sedation

Clinical assessment of sedation depth includes observation of loss of consciousness, snoring, and apnea.[9] Light sedation, defined as loss of response to verbal stimulation to a normal voice volume represents the best level of sedation when performing DISE. However, clinical assessment may be limited by the lack of standardization and reproducibility, making comparison between different centers more difficult.

Electroencephalogram (EEG)-derived parameters such as the Bispectral Index (BIS), spectral entropy, and qCON monitor are objective measurements of depth of sedation.[10] Of these 3 measures, the BIS is the most commonly used and published in literature. Unfortunately, there is still no universally acceptable level of BIS score target for DISE. De Vito and colleagues[5] recommended a target BIS range of 50 to 70 with a recommendation for more validation studies. It was a significant step and effort toward standardization of sedation monitoring. A later study by Lo and colleagues[11] demonstrated more upper airway collapse for a BIS of 50 to 60 (deep sedation) compared with a BIS of 65 to 75 (light sedation). However, it can be argued that the increase in airway collapsibility was more related to the sedating drug (propofol) than the BIS reading. Based on our observation, some patients may not be adequately sedated with BIS 65 to 75, making it not the perfect BIS target as well.

In a practical setting, we should combine both clinical assessment together with BIS monitoring to determine the best state for DISE. It should be the highest BIS level (within a standardized target range, eg, 50–70) when the patient is clinically sedated.

Drugs

Sedation is never exactly the same as natural sleep. The ideal drug should be able to achieve sedation that is similar to natural sleep with similar upper airway muscle tone. The 3 sedating drugs commonly used for DISE are midazolam, propofol, and dexmedetomidine, each one with its own advantages and disadvantages.

Midazolam, a benzodiazepine, was the first drug used in DISE. It was given in the form of boluses as described by Croft and Pringle in 1991.[4] However, midazolam is less commonly used nowadays because of its inconsistent mechanism of action, long duration of action, and difficulty achieving sedation that is comparable with a natural sleep state.[12]

Propofol is now the most commonly used sedating drug, replacing midazolam.[12] Anesthetists are familiar with propofol because it is a commonly used drug with well-known pharmacologic profile. It has a quick onset of action with short half-life, allowing rapid reversal from sedation within minutes. The sedation effect of propofol can achieve EEG profile that is similar to non–rapid eye movement sleep.[12] In a review of literature by Charakorn and Kezirian,[9] propofol sedation decreased the muscle tone of the genioglossus to a level between rapid eye movement and non–rapid eye movement sleep for normal subjects. However, it is also known to cause increased collapsibility of the upper airway in deeper sedation, which may lead to inaccuracy in the airway assessment.[13] Therefore, in the ideal situation upper airway evaluation should be interpreted with sedation depth using processed EEG parameters such as BIS.[13]

Dexmedetomidine is increasingly gaining popularity as an alternative to propofol for DISE. Like propofol, it is a commonly used drug by the anesthetist with relatively short half-life. Dexmedetomidine is able to sedate patients to a state similar to non–rapid eye movement sleep.[14] It also has some advantages over propofol because it causes less respiratory depression or decreases in upper airway tone. However, a significant proportion of patients may not be adequately sedated for DISE even at maximum dose (1.4 μg/kg/h).[15] **Table 1** illustrate the advantages and disadvantages of dexmedetomidine versus propofol based on Chang and colleagues's[16] systematic review. Although dexmedetomidine seems to be superior to propofol, it has its disadvantages and is often used in combination with other drugs, such as remifentanil or propofol to achieve the desired effects.[15]

In terms of method of administration and dosing strategies, there are many different techniques published in the literature that largely depends on the setting, staff, equipment, and drugs

Table 1
Advantages and disadvantages of dexmedetomidine versus propofol in DISE based on the systematic review by Chang and colleagues

	Dexmedetomidine	Propofol
Advantages	More stable sedation based on cardiorespiratory parameters Lower incidence of airway obstruction	Induces greater degree of upper airway collapse More reliable in achieving target depth of sedation Faster onset of action and shorter half-life
Disadvantages	May have inadequate upper airway collapse for DISE assessment Less reliable in achieving adequate sedation	Causes more respiratory depression Higher risk of more severe airway obstruction requiring intervention

Abbreviation: DISE, drug-induced sleep endoscopy.
Data from Chang ET, Certal V, Song SA, et al. Dexmedetomidine versus propofol during drug-induced sleep endoscopy and sedation: a systematic review. Sleep Breath 2017;21(3):727–35.

available. Atkins and Mandel[12] published an anesthesia review paper summarizing many different administration techniques and dosing strategies. The diverse published techniques include manual bolus, target-controlled infusion, infusion pump, probability ramp control, or a combination of the techniques.[12] A manual bolus gives the least predictable results with a higher risk of oversedation, worse desaturation, and less smooth transition to airway obstruction stage.[12] Slow administration with the lowest dose needed to achieve the target sedation effect should reduce the risk of complications. For example, De Vito and colleagues[5] recommended propofol dosing strategy using target-controlled infusion at a starting dose of 1.5 to 3.0 μg/mL with an increment rate of 0.2 to 0.5 until target is achieved. Overall, there remains a lack of universally acceptable drug of choice or administration technique for DISE. De Vito and colleagues[5] suggested a few possible dosing strategies that were agreeable by the European study group in 2014 and published in the European position paper on DISE.

EVALUATION OF UPPER AIRWAY COLLAPSE

Nasendoscopy can be performed when the patient is clinically sedated, ideally supported by objective EEG derivative such as BIS. Topical anesthetic to the nose and throat is not recommended because it may affect the upper airway reflex and reduce the upper airway dilator muscle tone.[17] De Vito and colleagues[5] recommended observation of at least 2 cycles of upper airway change with respiration for every level of the upper airway before documenting any airway collapse. The endoscopy can be done with the patient in different positions depending on the preference of the clinician. It is frequently done in the supine position because it is a common sleep position with OSA at its worst.[9] Assessment with head rotation (body in supine) is similar to the head and body in a lateral position in the level, severity, and configuration of upper airway collapse, except for the velum (less severe anteroposterior collapse in head rotation alone).[18] A manual jaw advancement can also be done during DISE and may be useful in predicting the effect of a MAD.[19] **Figs. 1–4** demonstrate various patterns of upper airway collapse at different levels.

Flexible endoscopy is performed through the nasal cavity, observing every level of the upper airway until the larynx. There is no universally accepted grading system to document the upper airway collapse during DISE. The Pringle and Croft[20] grading system was the first classification

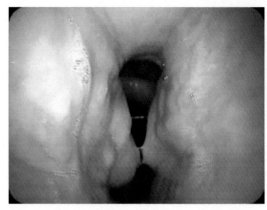

Fig. 1. Lateral oropharyngeal narrowing secondary to tonsillar hypertrophy.

described in 1993. The Pringle and Croft classification was commonly used in earlier studies published before 2007.[6] Since then, many new classifications were described by different institutions all over the world. Based on a literature review, the 3 most common classification used were the velum oropharynx, tongue base, epiglottis (VOTE) system (38.6%), Pringle and Croft grading (15.9%), and the nose oropharynx hypopharynx larynx (NOHL) system (9.1%).[6] The European position paper on DISE recommended a scoring system that documents the level (and/or structure), degree (severity), and configuration (pattern, direction) of obstruction.[5] The VOTE[21] and NOHL[22] systems are the 2 most common for grading that fulfill the criteria recommended. **Table 2** summarizes the VOTE and NOHL classification systems.

The VOTE and NOHL classifications have some similarities and are both relatively simple to learn and easy to apply. The NOHL system may

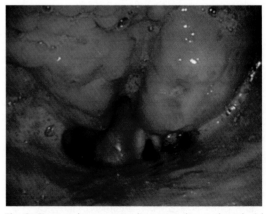

Fig. 2. Tongue base narrowing secondary to lymphoid hypertrophy.

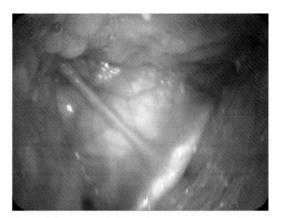

Fig. 3. Primary epiglottic collapse.

have some advantages because it describes an additional level of obstruction in the nose and can be used in both awake and sleep endoscopy. However, a small study comparing VOTE and NOHL in DISE noted that the VOTE grading system was more comprehensive in the evaluation of the pharynx and epiglottis.[23]

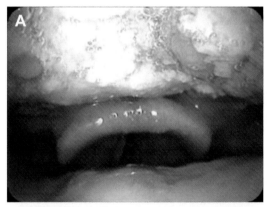

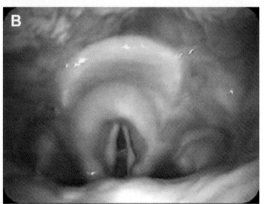

Fig. 4. (*A*) Hypopharynx and epiglottis in supine position. (*B*) Hypopharynx and larynx with manual jaw advancement.

CLINICAL APPLICATION FOR TREATMENT OPTIONS SELECTION
Surgery

The surgical treatment options for OSA are usually determined by the following:

a. Patient factors: Awake and DISE upper airway evaluation, severity of OSA, body mass index, and medical comorbidities.
b. Surgeon factors: Surgeon's training and preferred surgical techniques.
c. Equipment and facilities: The availability of surgical instruments (eg, surgical robot, coblator or radiofrequency devices) and the facilities to provide close monitoring after surgery for OSA.

It is well-known that the upper airway of patients with OSA changes from the awake to sleep state. In a systematic review of literature, more than 50% of the planned OSA surgeries (based on awake examination) were modified after DISE.[24] The change in surgery were mainly owing to the difference in hypopharyngeal or laryngeal obstruction in DISE compared with awake endoscopy.[24]

Overall, there remains a lack of literature to associate DISE with improved surgical outcomes.[24] In a small, retrospective study by Soares and colleagues,[25] DISE findings of significant lateral oropharyngeal wall collapse and/or supraglottic collapse were associated with higher risk of surgical failure. Transoral robotic surgery may be able to address the supraglottic obstruction for primary epiglottic collapse or epiglottic collapse secondary to tongue base obstruction.[26] However, transoral robotic surgery with or without multilevel surgery is likely to work only in patients with no significant lateral oropharyngeal wall collapse.[27] Therefore, DISE is useful to identify potential surgical candidates among patients with OSA.

Upper Airway Stimulation

Hypoglossal nerve stimulation of the upper airway is a new promising treatment modality for OSA. The Stimulation Therapy for Apnea Reduction (STAR) trial is an ongoing prospective cohort study with a very strict patient selection criteria for upper airway stimulation therapy that includes DISE.[28] The absence of complete concentric collapse of the soft palate during DISE is associated with a better treatment outcome.[29] Therefore, DISE is an important assessment tool to help identify suitable patients for upper airway stimulation therapy.

Mandibular Advancement Device

A MAD is a well-recognized treatment option for patients with mild to moderate OSA. Manual jaw

Table 2
Comparison of VOTE and NOHL classification in the grading of upper airway collapse in DISE

Classification	VOTE[21]	NOHL[22]

Level/structure	Velum
	Oropharynx (lateral oropharyngeal wall)
	Tongue base
	Epiglottis
		Nose
		Oropharynx
		Hypopharynx
		Larynx
		  Supraglottis
		  Glottis

Grade of collapse	0—No obstruction (no vibration) 1—Partial obstruction (vibration) 2—Complete obstruction (collapse) X—Not visualized	Nose, oropharynx and hypopharynx: 1—0%–25% 2—25%–50% 3—50%–75% 4—75%–100% Larynx—Positive or negative
Configuration of collapse	AP, lateral, and circular	AP, lateral and circular

Abbreviations: AP, anteroposterior; DISE, drug-induced sleep endoscopy; NOHL, nose oropharynx hypopharynx and larynx; VOTE, velum oropharynx, tongue base, epiglottis.

advancement by about 5 mm during DISE may simulate the potential effect of MAD.[19] Patients with good improvement in upper airway patency during manual jaw advancement are more likely to benefit from MAD therapy.[19] To further improve the accuracy of DISE MAD simulation, a custom-made simulation bite in maximum comfortable protrusion (pretested and calculated when awake) can be applied during DISE.[30] A significant improvement in upper airway with simulation bite is associated with better treatment outcome with MAD.[30]

Positional Therapy

Positional therapy is an effective treatment option for patients with positional OSA. Positional OSA is diagnosed when a patient has apnea–hypopnea index of more than 5, with a supine apnea–hypopnea index of at least 2 times that of nonsupine.[31] The diagnosis of positional OSA may be missed if a patient sleeps in pure supine position or when there is a lack of recording of sleep position during a sleep study. For this group of patients with OSA, DISE in different sleep positions may identify those who can benefit from positional therapy. Patients with positional OSA will likely have at least partial improvement in upper airway patency in a lateral sleep position.[32] Head rotation (with body in supine) during DISE is also more effective in improving upper airway patency for positional OSA compared with non-positional OSA patient.[33] Therefore, a patient with improvement in upper airway patency in non-supine position will likely benefit from positional therapy.

FUTURE DIRECTIONS

It is difficult to directly compare the heterogeneous published literature on DISE from different centers across the world. There should be some consensus on the standardization for DISE sedation drugs and technique, monitoring of sedation depth, and classification of the upper airway collapse. So far, the European position paper on DISE[5] group has made several recommendations in the effort to standardize DISE. The group also noted the need for validation studies for different aspects of DISE.[5] With the large number of recent literature on DISE, the sleep centers around the world should work together in the near future to come out with some standardization for a DISE technique and have some consensus on a universally acceptable classification system for upper airway evaluation.

SUMMARY

DISE is a safe and practical technique to evaluate the dynamic upper airway collapse during sleep. It is proven to be useful in the treatment options selection for patients with OSA. Although DISE is commonly used to assist surgical decision making, there remains a lack of literature to associate DISE with improved surgical outcomes. Owing to the lack of standardization for DISE, it is difficult to compare the published literature across different sleep centers.

REFERENCES

1. Trudo FJ, Gefter WB, Welch KC, et al. State-related changes in upper airway caliber and surrounding

soft- tissue structures in normal subjects. Am J Respir Crit Care Med 1998;158(4):1259–70.

2. Friedman M, Salapatas AM, Bonzelaar LB. Updated Friedman staging system for obstructive sleep apnea. Adv Otorhinolaryngol 2017;80:41–8.

3. Borowiecki B, Pollak CP, Weitzman ED, et al. Fibrooptic study of pharyngeal airway during sleep in patients with hypersomnia obstructive sleep apnea syndrome. Laryngoscope 1978;88(8):1310–3.

4. Croft CB, Pringle M. Sleep nasendoscopy: a technique of assessment in snoring and obstructive sleep apnoea. Clin Otolaryngol Allied Sci 1991; 16(5):504–9.

5. De Vito A, Carrasco Llatas M, Vanni A, et al. European position paper on drug-induced sedation endoscopy (DISE). Sleep Breath 2014;18(3):453–65.

6. Amos JM, Durr ML, Nardone HC, et al. Systematic review of drug-induced sleep endoscopy scoring systems. Otolaryngol Head Neck Surg 2018; 158(2):240–8.

7. Vanderveken OM. Drug-induced sleep endoscopy (DISE) for non-CPAP treatment selection in patients with sleep-disordered breathing. Sleep Breath 2013;17(1):13–4.

8. Kezirian EJ. Nonresponders to pharyngeal surgery for obstructive sleep apnea: insights from drug-induced sleep endoscopy. Laryngoscope 2011; 121(6):1320–6.

9. Charakorn N, Kezirian EJ. Drug-induced sleep endoscopy. Otolaryngol Clin North Am 2016;49(6): 1359–72.

10. Müller JN, Kreuzer M, García PS, et al. Monitoring depth of sedation: evaluating the agreement between the Bispectral Index, qCON and the Entropy Module's State Entropy during flexible bronchoscopy. Minerva Anestesiol 2017;83(6):563–73.

11. Lo YL, Ni YL, Wang TY, et al. Bispectral index in evaluating effects of sedation depth on drug-induced sleep endoscopy. J Clin Sleep Med 2015;11(9): 1011–20.

12. Atkins JH, Mandel JE. Drug-induced sleep endoscopy: from obscure technique to diagnostic tool for assessment of obstructive sleep apnea for surgical interventions. Curr Opin Anaesthesiol 2018;31(1): 120–6.

13. Kellner P, Herzog B, Plößl S, et al. Depth-dependent changes of obstruction patterns under increasing sedation during drug-induced sedation endoscopy: results of a German monocentric clinical trial. Sleep Breath 2016;20(3):1035–43.

14. Huupponen E, Maksimow A, Lapinlampi P, et al. Electroencephalogram spindle activity during dexmedetomidine sedation and physiological sleep. Acta Anaesthesiol Scand 2008;52(2):289–94.

15. Cho JS, Soh S, Kim EJ, et al. Comparison of three sedation regimens for drug-induced sleep endoscopy. Sleep Breath 2015;19(2):711–7.

16. Chang ET, Certal V, Song SA, et al. Dexmedetomidine versus propofol during drug-induced sleep endoscopy and sedation: a systematic review. Sleep Breath 2017;21(3):727–35.

17. Fogel RB, Malhotra A, Shea SA, et al. Reduced genioglossal activity with upper airway anesthesia in awake patients with OSA. J Appl Physiol (1985) 2000;88(4):1346–54.

18. Safiruddin F, Koutsourelakis I, de Vries N. Upper airway collapse during drug induced sleep endoscopy: head rotation in supine position compared with lateral head and trunk position. Eur Arch Oto-rhino-laryngology 2014;272(2):485–8.

19. Johal A, Hector MP, Battagel JM, et al. Impact of sleep nasendoscopy on the outcome of mandibular advancement splint therapy in subjects with sleep-related breathing disorders. J Laryngol Otol 2007; 121(7):668–75.

20. Pringle MB, Croft CB. A grading system for patients with obstructive sleep apnoea-based on sleep nasendoscopy. Clin Otolaryngol Allied Sci 1993; 18(6):480–4. Available at: http://www.ncbi.nlm.nih. gov/pubmed/8877224. Accessed February 12, 2018.

21. Kezirian EJ, Hohenhorst W, De Vries N. Drug-induced sleep endoscopy: the VOTE classification. Eur Arch Otorhinolaryngol 2011;268(8):1233–6.

22. Vicini C, De Vito A, Benazzo M, et al. The nose oropharynx hypopharynx and larynx (NOHL) classification: a new system of diagnostic standardized examination for OSAHS patients. Eur Arch Otorhinolaryngol 2012;269(4):1297–300.

23. da Cunha Viana A, Mendes DL, de Andrade Lemes LN, et al. Drug-induced sleep endoscopy in the obstructive sleep apnea: comparison between NOHL and VOTE classifications. Eur Arch Otorhinolaryngol 2017;274(2):627–35.

24. Certal VF, Pratas R, Guimaraes L, et al. Awake examination versus DISE for surgical decision making in patients with OSA: a systematic review. Laryngoscope 2016;126(3):768–74.

25. Soares D, Sinawe H, Folbe AJ, et al. Lateral oropharyngeal wall and supraglottic airway collapse associated with failure in sleep apnea surgery. Laryngoscope 2012;122(2):473–9.

26. Vicini C, Montevecchi F, Tenti G, et al. Transoral robotic surgery: tongue base reduction and supraglottoplasty for obstructive sleep apnea. Oper Tech Otolaryngol - Head Neck Surg 2012;23(1): 45–7.

27. Meraj TS, Muenz DG, Glazer TA, et al. Does drug-induced sleep endoscopy predict surgical success in transoral robotic multilevel surgery in obstructive sleep apnea? Laryngoscope 2017; 127(4):971–6.

28. Strollo PJ, Gillespie MB, Soose RJ, et al. Upper airway stimulation for obstructive sleep

apnea: durability of the treatment effect at 18 months. Sleep 2015;38(10):1593–8.

29. Vanderveken OM, Maurer JT, Hohenhorst W, et al. Evaluation of drug-induced sleep endoscopy as a patient selection tool for implanted upper airway stimulation for obstructive sleep apnea. J Clin Sleep Med 2013;9(5):433–8.

30. Vroegop AVMT, Vanderveken OM, Dieltjens M, et al. Sleep endoscopy with simulation bite for prediction of oral appliance treatment outcome. J Sleep Res 2013;22(3):348–55.

31. Lloyd SR, Cartwright RD. Physiologic basis of therapy for sleep apnea. Am Rev Respir Dis 1987; 136(2):525–6.

32. Victores AJ, Hamblin J, Gilbert J, et al. Usefulness of sleep endoscopy in predicting positional obstructive sleep apnea. Otolaryngol Head Neck Surg 2014; 150:487–93.

33. Safiruddin F, Koutsourelakis I, De Vries N. Analysis of the influence of head rotation during drug-induced sleep endoscopy in obstructive sleep apnea. Laryngoscope 2014;124(9):2195–9.

Establishing a Patent Nasal Passage in Obstructive Sleep Apnea

Chiba Shintaro, MD, PhD[a], Chan-Soon Park, MD, PhD[b],*

KEYWORDS

- Nose • Sleep-disordered breathing • Airway resistance • CPAP • Allergic rhinitis

KEY POINTS

- Nose may not be a passive but an active noncollapsible tube to participate in the pathophysiology of sleep-disordered breathing.
- Nasal treatment might not reduce OSA severity (apnea-hypopnea index [AHI]) significantly or less effectively than expected.
- The roles of nasal treatments for OSA are not only the reduction of AHI, but also the improvement of subjective symptoms and sleep quality, including CPAP adherence.

INTRODUCTION

Sleep-disordered breathing (SDB) means a wide range of chronic breathing problems during sleep from flow limitation to sleep apnea, obstructive (OSA) or central (CSA). OSA is usually described as repeated episodes of partial or complete cessation of airflow during sleep.

SDB causes recurrent hypoxia, altered autonomic nervous system activity, and fluctuation of blood pressure during sleep, so patients with SDB are closely related to a wide range of diseases and problems, such as hypertension, cerebrovascular accidents, traffic accidents, and daily functioning.

According to the study by Peppard and colleagues,[1] the prevalence of moderate to severe SDB in the United States is 10% among 30-year-old to 49-year-old men; 17% among 50-year-old to 70-year-old men; 3% among 30-year-old to 49-year-old women; and 9% among 50-year-old to 70-year-old women, which showed substantial increases over the past 2 decades.

Although SDB is a common disorder globally, the pathophysiology and mechanisms of SDB have not been fully elucidated, in which the role of the nose has been ignored or underestimated.

However, considering that the nose makes more than 50% of the total resistance of the upper airway and nasal breathing is the physiologic respiratory route for breathing during sleep, the nose might take more part in the pathophysiology and mechanisms of SDB. The nose also serves a variety of physiologic functions, such as olfaction, humidification, heating of air, and filtration.[2–4]

Repeated partial (flow limitation, hypopnea) or complete (apnea) airway obstruction and increased respiratory effort could be caused by a mismatch among factors to maintain upper airway patency, like anatomic, neuromuscular, and

Conflicts of Interest: The author has no financial conflicts of interest.

The pathophysiology part of this article is partially based on an article published by Sleep Med Res (2014;5(1): 1–4), which was written by C.-S. Park.

[a] Department of Otorhinolaryngology–Head and Neck Surgery, Jikei University School of Medicine, Tokyo, 105-8461 Japan; [b] Department of Otorhinolaryngology–Head and Neck Surgery, St Vincent's Hospital, College of Medicine, The Catholic University of Korea, 93 Jungbu-daero, Paldal-gu, Suwon City, Gyeonggi Province, 16247 Republic of Korea

* Corresponding author.

E-mail address: pcs0112@catholic.ac.kr

Sleep Med Clin 14 (2019) 41–50

https://doi.org/10.1016/j.jsmc.2018.10.005

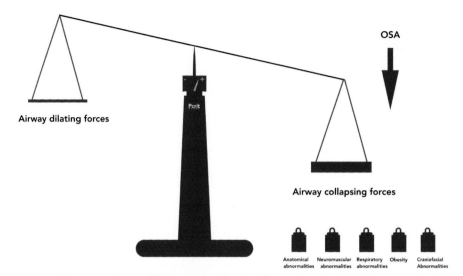

Fig. 1. The balance between airway dilating and collapsing forces in SDB. Pcrit, Pharyngeal critical pressure. (*Adapted from* Park CS. Role of nose in sleep-disordered breathing. Sleep Med Res 2014;5(1):2; with permission.)

respiratory factors, which are harmonious in subjects without SDB (**Fig. 1**).

To date, in the pathogenesis of SDB, the nose has been regarded as a noncollapsible nonfunctioning tube, as described in the Staring resistor model (**Fig. 2**).

However, recent studies showed that the nose might not be a nonfunctioning or passive tube in the pathogenesis of SDB, and the nose might be related to the collapsibility of the remaining upper airway.

The efficiency of nasal treatment for OSA still remains controversial. To date, many studies indicated that nasal treatment can improve subjective symptoms related to OSA and quality of life, but the effect to decrease objective parameters like AHI has not been consistent.

This article aims to review the role of the nose on the pathogenesis of SDB and the meaning of nasal treatment on SDB.

THE ROLE OF NASAL BREATHING ON SLEEP-DISORDERED BREATHING: FROM THE ANATOMIC POINTS OF VIEW

Nasal obstruction as a potential risk factor for OSA syndrome (OSAS) has been reported in many articles.[5,6] Especially a study by Young and colleagues[7] found that nasal obstruction was an independent contributor to OSAS.

Nasal obstruction can have a negative effect on respiration because nasal breathing is more efficient than mouth breathing, especially during sleep.

In addition, the postural change during sleep can aggravate nasal obstruction much more,

which might be caused by postural reflex mechanisms and the changes of hydrostatic pressure on nasal venous circulation.[8–10]

Virkkula and colleagues[11] showed that nasal resistance, especially in the supine position, was related to sleep parameters in nonobese patients.

Considering Poiseuille's law, which means that resistance to airflow varies with the fourth power of the radius, there are many conditions, anatomic abnormalities, and diseases to decrease the radius of nasal cavity and then increase nasal resistance.

Nasal airway resistance was shown to be linearly correlated to the apnea-hypopnea index (AHI), which might mean any condition or disease to increase nasal airway resistance could cause SDB.[12]

Sleep apnea and frequent arousal were also reported to be related to nasal obstruction, because nasal obstruction might increase nasal resistance and then cause more negative oropharyngeal pressure during inspiration.[13–15]

Considering these factors, nasal obstruction may predispose to upper airway collapse.

THE ROLE OF NASAL BREATHING ON SLEEP-DISORDERED BREATHING: FROM THE NEUROMUSCULAR POINT OF VIEW

The mucosal V3 afferents are known to be responsible for the trigemino-hypoglossal reflex via the dorsal part of the trigeminal principal sensory nucleus to hypoglossal motoneurones.[16]

The mechanoreceptors of the upper airway are known to play important roles in reflex against negative pressure of the upper airway because

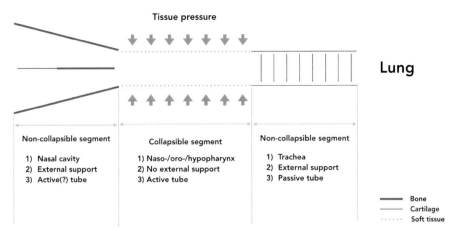

Fig. 2. Starling resistor model. (*Adapted from* Park CS. Role of nose in sleep-disordered breathing. Sleep Med Res 2014;5(1):3; with permission.)

the reflex activation of genioglossus muscle is modulated by input signal from mechanoreceptors in the airway.[17]

The change of intraluminal pressure or airflow during inspiration may stimulate mechanoreceptors, which may send afferent signals to the nucleus solitary tract in the medulla, and then via the hypoglossal motor neuron, may change the activity of the genioglossus muscle.[18]

Nasal obstruction can cause mouth opening and breathing, which can cause dryness of the mouth and might lower the sensitivity of the V3 afferent. Mechanical vibration, such as snoring, may cause trauma to upper airway, which might also lower the sensitivity of V3 afferent.

Although it has not been shown that the nasal mechanoreceptor innervated by maxillary nerve (V2) might be directly related to mechanoreceptor reflex of upper airway muscles, including genioglossus muscle, like mandibular nerve or superior laryngeal nerve, there have been only a few studies on the existence of nasal mechanoreceptors responsive to airflow and SDB.

Wallois and colleagues[19] reported that trigeminal nasal receptors related to respiration or air jet within the nasal cavity were found in the ethmoidal nerve in cats.

A study showed that the nasal vestibule is twice as sensitive as the nasal cavum to an air jet at mean intranasal temperature and that the nasal vestibule is very sensitive to the tactile stimulation of an air jet.[20]

Anesthesia of the vestibule was also shown to decrease nasal sensation of airflow by Aldren and Tolley,[21] which meant there were mechanoreceptors to airflow around the nasal vestibule.

White and colleagues[22] reported that anesthesia of the nasal passages caused sleep apnea in 10

healthy men during sleep, and the magnitude of these changes is similar to that previously reported with complete nasal obstruction. So, the investigators concluded that nasal receptors sensitive to air flow may be important in maintaining breathing rhythmicity during sleep.

Considering these factors, although there was no report showing the direct connection between the mucosal maxillary nerve (cranial nerve V2) and hypoglossal nerve, it is clear that there are nasal mechanoreceptors responsive to air flow or pressure and decreased sensitivities of nasal mechanoreceptors by any cause might be related to abnormal breathing during sleep.

According to Jordan and colleagues,[23] compensatory mechanisms (increased genioglossus muscle activity and/or duty cycle) during sleep against partial upper airway collapse or pressure change may be less effective in obese patients with OSA than in non-snorers. Although all compensatory mechanisms cannot be explained by nasal mechanoreceptors, the nose may play a partial role in compensatory mechanisms with, for example, obesity or neuropathy.

THE ROLE OF NASAL BREATHING ON SLEEP-DISORDERED BREATHING: FROM THE RESPIRATORY POINTS OF VIEW

According to the classic Starling resistor model, the airway is usually divided into 3 segments: non-collapsible nasal and tracheal segments and a collapsible pharyngeal segment.[24]

The balance between airway dilating and collapsing forces is critical to maintain airway patency. If disturbed, the airway may collapse partially or completely.[24]

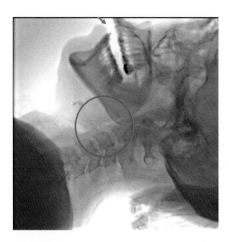 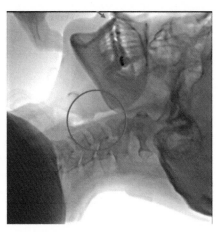

Mouth opened, supine position   Mouth closed, supine position

Fig. 3. The difference of airway size (circle, small [Left] or large [Right]) according to the state of mouth (arrow, opened [Left] or closed [Right]) on videofluoro scopy during sleep induced with midazolam.

The nasal cavity is a noncollapsible tube due to rigid support by bone but not a passive tube as described in the Starling resistor model.

The nasal turbinate mucosa is actively responsive to temperature, humidity, emotion, diseases, and so on, which means the nose can change total airway resistance.

If the narrowest cross-sectional area of the nose by any cause is changed, the velocity of airflow after this point can be changed (like the Venturi effect), which might cause the change in airflow pressure, stimulate nasal mechanoreceptors, and finally modulate the collapsibility of the upper airway.

Another point to be considered is air flow in the nose, laminar flow. If the laminar flow of the nose is converted to turbulent flow, nasal mucosa will be dried up and its mechanoreceptors will not function well. Many nasal deformities and diseases can convert nasal laminar to turbulent flow, such as turbinate hypertrophy, nasal polyp, and septal deviation.

The other point is nasal obstruction causing mouth breathing, which is not a physiologic breathing route during sleep.

Patients with nasal obstruction are obliged to choose mouth breathing to secure ventilation, but mouth breathing causes the jaw and hyoid bone (including tongue) to move downward and backward, which can finally narrow the upper airway (**Fig. 3**).

Therefore, mouth breathers may be predisposed to upper airway collapse and SDB. This might be supported by the findings that the proportion of nasal breathing epochs preoperatively can accurately delineate the subgroup of patients who can benefit from nasal surgery.[25]

Therefore, reeducation and restoration of nasal breathing by upper airway myofunctional therapy might be important after any nasal or other treatments in patients with SDB.

THE EFFECTS OF NASAL TREATMENTS ON OBSTRUCTIVE SLEEP APNEA

It is said that the nasal airway is the original and preferred delivery route. As described previously, nasal obstructions due to anatomic abnormalities and inflammatory diseases are associated with increased risk of snoring, OSA, reduced sleep quality, and increased daytime sleepiness. Furthermore, nasal obstruction reduced continuous positive airway pressure (CPAP) adherence.

Primary anatomic abnormalities are septal deviation and hypertrophied turbinates. Common inflammatory diseases include rhinitis (allergic and nonallergic), sinusitis, and polyps.

The prevalence of nasal obstruction is unknown; however, prevalence of these nasal diseases in patients with OSA is expected more than 30%.

Drug Therapy

The *Cochrane Database of Systematic Reviews* in 2006 concluded that there is insufficient evidence to recommend the use of drug therapy in the treatment of OSA.[26] Small studies have reported positive effects of topical application of sympathomimetic vasoconstrictors (eg, xylometazoline) or topical nasal steroids on short-term outcome.[27,28] Data from these studies suggest that pharmacologically induced improvement of nasal patency in patients with OSA has some beneficial effects on the severity of OSA and on sleep architecture.

Nasal Dilator

There are some studies that nasal dilators improve nasal patency, which results in a reduction of snoring events, but they seem to have an only minor effect on OSA severity and symptoms.[29–32] One interesting study concluded that an external nasal dilator reduces arousal instability in snorers without OSA using cyclic alternating pattern (CAP) analysis.[33]

Nasal Surgery

The efficiency of nasal surgery for OSA remains controversial. Two meta-analyses and other articles on this topic indicated that nasal surgery can improve subjective sleepiness (Epworth Sleepiness Scale [ESS] score) and quality of life.[34–47]

However, objective evaluation of OSA severity (AHI) did not reduce significantly. On the other hand, one meta-analysis and others said nasal surgery can improve not only daytime sleepiness but also decrease AHI.[48–54]

Morinaga and colleagues[37] reported that milder OSA, lower body mass index (BMI), and normal preoperative cephalometry have also been proposed to be factors favoring improvement in OSA severity from nasal surgery.

In any case, the surgical reduction of nasal resistance led to improved sleep quality, decreased snoring, and reduced daytime sleepiness despite no significant changes in AHI.

Fig. 4 shows the results of our small study about polysomnograph (PSG) parameter change including CAP in 15 patients with OSA (14 men, 1 woman: median age: 44 years old, median BMI: 25.4 kg/m^2, median AHI: 31.7 episodes per hour) who received nasal surgery.

After surgery, AHI, Arousal Index, sleep efficiency, %stage1, %stageSWS (slow wave sleep), and %stageREM (rapid eye movement) did not change, but CAP rate decreased significantly from 40.67% to 32.02%.

CAP (29) is a spontaneous rhythm of non-REM sleep characterized by electroencephalogram oscillations corresponding to recurrent activation events and unstable sleep depth. CAP analysis shows high sensitivity in the detection of sleep disorders than the method that we used conventionally, and now considered to be a comprehensive tool to study sleep instability. Because CAP rate is known to be related to subjective sleep quality (visual analog scale), from our results, it can be inferred that the improvement of nasal obstruction by surgery lead sleep stability despite no significant changes in AHI and other sleep parameters after nasal surgery (**Table 1**).

CONTINUOUS POSITIVE AIRWAY PRESSURE ADHERENCE AND NASAL SURGERY

Nasal CPAP therapy is considered the first-line therapy for moderate-severe OSA. CPAP is highly efficacious but the adherence rate is not high (30). Nasal obstruction is a common complaint among CPAP users, with an estimated prevalence of 25% to 45%.[55–57]

In the SAVE study, CPAP use at 1 month and side effects at 1 month were the only independent predictors of 12-month CPAP adherence. CPAP side effects include dry mouth, nasal symptoms, and mask fit or leak problems. Many of these complaints are associated with the level of CPAP pressure, with higher pressures associated with reduced CPAP adherence.[58]

Nasal surgery improves the nasal resistance and reduced optimal positive airway pressure (PAP) pressure. And also, another predictors of PAP adherence is the change of daytime sleepiness (ESS) from baseline to 1 month.

Tagaya and colleagues (35) reported that the comparison of nasal surgery and CPAP on daytime sleepiness in patients with OSAS and concluded nasal surgery is more satisfactory for

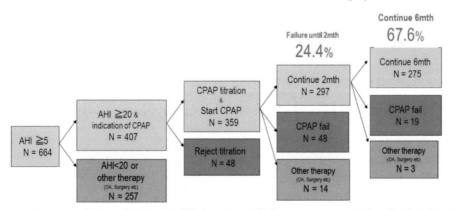

Fig. 4. Six month course of the patients with OSA to whom CPAP was recommended as the first-line therapy.

Table 1
Polysomnography parameters before and after nasal surgery

	Pretreatment	Post Surgery	P
TST, min	393.25	397.5	.72989
Sleep latency, min	8	7.25	.77756
REM_latency, min	72.25	81.25	.50980
SE, %	85.7	86.95	.20917
STAGE1, %	27.6	32.2	.57199
STAGE2, %	47.9	46.2	.92498
SWS, %	0.75	0.15	.85895
REM, %	18.85	18.75	.85058
AHI, /h	34.25	33.35	.45115
NREM_AHI, /h	37.5	30.45	.24549
REM_AHI, /h	36.65	42.85	.68324
OD <90%, %	1.15	0.65	.294
ODI <3%, %	16.75	20.15	.47034
Arousal index	29.3	30.1	.63768
CAP rate	40.67	32.02	.035

Change of Sleep structure before and after nasal surgery on 15 OSA. After surgery, AHI, Arousal Index, sleep efficiency, %stage1, %stageSWS, and %stageREM did not change, but CAP rate decreased significantly from 40.67% to 32.02%.

Abbreviations: AHI, apnea-hypopnea index; CAP, cyclic alternating pattern; NREM, non-rapid eye movement; OD, oxygen desaturation; ODI, oxygen desaturation index; REM, rapid eye movement; SE, sleep efficiency; SWS, slow wave sleep; TST, total sleep time.

some patients with OSAS than CPAP on daytime sleepiness.[59]

A general, OSA outcomes assessment by American academy of sleep medicine guidelines includes resolution of sleepiness, OSA-specific quality-of-life measures, patient and spousal satisfaction, adherence to therapy, avoidance of factors worsening disease, obtaining an adequate amount of sleep, practicing proper sleep hygiene, and weight loss for overweight/obese patients.[60] Nasal surgery is known not only to reduce CPAP, but also to improve daytime sleepiness, subjective sleep quality, and sleep-related quality of life measure.

So it can be said that nasal surgery plays a key adjunctive role in the management of CPAP adherence.

HOW MANY AND WHICH PATIENTS WOULD REQUIRE NASAL TREATMENT?

Nasal obstruction has big impact of CPAP adherence through increasing PAP pressure and worth daytime sleepiness. Therefore, it is necessary to treat any nasal obstruction before initiating CPAP. But the indication or criteria of nasal treatment for CPAP users is still unclear.

In our prospective study about nasal resistance versus CPAP adherence, 664 consecutive patients with OSA diagnosed by PSG were enrolled. **Fig. 5** shows 6-month course of the patients with OSA who recommended CPAP therapy as first-line treatment. Finally, 67.6% patients continued CPAP therapy (see **Fig. 4**).

Results were as follows:

1. 24.4% (96 of 407) rejected CPAP titration or stopped Nasal continuous positive airway pressure (nCPAP) therapy within 2 months. Nasal resistance in the early CPAP failure group (failed within 2 months) is significantly higher than that of the CPAP-tolerant group (0.26 pa/cm^3/s vs 0.22 pa/cm^3/s; 100 pa) (see **Fig. 5**A).
2. 30.1% (108 of 359) require nasal therapy when using nCPAP. There was statistical difference in the nasal resistance between the patients with nasal treatment and the patients without (0.26 pa/cm^3/s vs 0.21pa/cm^3/s; 100 pa, P = .002) (see **Fig. 5**B).
3. Finally, 9.3% (41 of 407) received nasal surgery (deviatomy, conchotomy).

From these data using multivariate regression analysis, it was found that the independent predictors of nasal treatment necessity in CPAP users are allergic rhinitis (AR) (odds ratio = 7.76, P<.00), sinusitis (odds ratio = 3.61, P<.00), and nasal resistance >0.30 pa/cm^3/s (odds ratio = 3.95, P<.03). On the other hand, the independent predictors of nasal surgery necessity in CPAP users are AR (odds ratio = 7.21, P<.00), ratio of the bilateral nasal cross section >3.0 (odds ratio = 2.83, P<.04).

With our results, we can predict the PAP patients who require nasal treatment or surgery before starting CPAP therapy.

ALLERGIC RHINITIS AND ITS UNIQUE IMPACT ON SLEEP

AR is a type 1 hypersensitivity reaction of the nasal mucosa mediated by immunoglobulin (Ig)E and T helper 2 (TH2) cells in response to inhaled environmental allergens.[61] Rhinitis is a common problem that causes disabilities worldwide. In industrialized countries, AR affects approximately 10% to 30% of the population with various prevalence rates according to recent studies.[62,63] The most commonly reported symptom of AR is nasal obstruction.[64,65] Nasal obstruction also has been shown to increase upper airway resistance and play a role in OSAS.[66] In addition to nasal obstruction, systemic release of mediators of AR such as

Nasal resistance
(pa/cm³/sec)

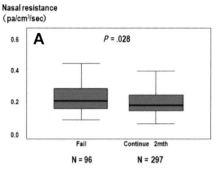

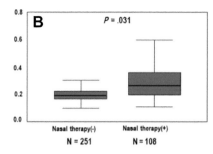

Fig. 5. (A) The difference of nasal resistance between CPAP failure and CPAP-tolerant groups. (B) The difference of nasal resistance between patients with and without nasal therapy.

inflammatory cytokines and histamine may lead to decreased cognition and arousal, as well as daytime somnolence.[67,68] A recent article showed that AR influences sleep more than expected, and a sleep disorder due to AR may influence symptoms in the daytime function including daytime sleepiness.[69]

However, details of the association between AR and sleep disorders are still unclear.

The first report using an objective evaluation on the sleep and breathing of patients with AR was carried out by Lavie and others.[70] Increase of nasal resistance due to AR increased micro-arousal on electroencephalogram, and they reported that the nasal resistance also influenced sleep. Furthermore, Young and others[71] pointed out that nasal obstruction was a factor in OSA during sleep, as shown by an epidemiologic investigation. As a result, sleep fragmentation caused by OSA may result in daytime sleepiness. There is also a report that nasal obstruction influences sleep or sleepiness on its own. Udaka and colleagues[72] and Hiraki and colleagues[73] showed that nasal obstruction without snoring influences sleepiness. Furthermore, nasal obstruction without AR influences sleepiness. In other words, these studies suggest that sleepiness may be directly related to nasal obstruction, and not just because of sleep apnea, as previously believed.

In addition to nasal obstruction, systemic release of mediators of AR, such as inflammatory cytokines and histamine, may influence the sleep/wake center directly, and lead to decreased cognition and arousal, as well as daytime somnolence. Krouse (43) and colleagues[67] report that Plasma interleukin (IL)1β, IL4, and IL10 rise in patients with AR, and that REM sleep decreases.

As for the reason why AR influences sleep, these 3 following hypotheses are presented:

1. Nasal obstruction due to AR causes OSA, and, as a result, a sleep disorder causes sleepiness.

2. Directly, nasal obstruction is related to sleepiness by obstructing the quality of the sleep (regardless of OSA).
3. Allergic disease by itself influences the sleep/wake center (through an inflammatory mediator) and causes a sleep disorder and sleepiness.

All these hypotheses may further be affected by changes in brain chemistry due to circadian rhythm.

Clearly, the relationship among nasal obstruction, allergic disease, sleep disorders, OSAS, inflammatory mediators, and the sleep/wake center is not yet clear.

We should consider not only influence of nasal obstruction on OSA, but also the impact of specific allergic pathophysiology on sleep/wake regulation.

SUMMARY

The nose accounts for more than 50% of the total resistance of the upper airway and is a physiologic breathing route during sleep.

In contrast to the explanation of the classic Staring resistor model, the nose may play more important roles in upper airway collapse during sleep and is not simply a passive tube.

From the anatomic, neuromuscular, and respiratory points of views, the role of the nose on airflow must be considered in patients with SDB and their treatments.

Nasal treatment could not reduce OSA severity directly; however, it is thought that nasal treatment has a key role in total management strategy for OSA as one airway from nose to larynx. The roles of nasal treatments for OSA are not only the reduction of AHI, but also the improvement of subjective symptoms and sleep quality, including CPAP adherence.

REFERENCES

1. Peppard PE, Young T, Barnet JH, et al. Increased prevalence of sleep-disordered breathing in adults. Am J Epidemiol 2013;177(9):1006–14.

2. Churchill SE, Shackelford LL, Georgi JN, et al. Morphological variation and airflow dynamics in the human nose. Am J Hum Biol 2004;16(6):625–38.

3. Ferris BG Jr, Mead J, Opie LH. Partitioning of respiratory flow resistance in man. J Appl Physiol 1964; 19:653–8.

4. Proctor DF. The upper airways. I. Nasal physiology and defense of the lungs. Am Rev Respir Dis 1977;115(1):97–129.

5. McNicholas WT, Tarlo S, Cole P, et al. Obstructive apneas during sleep in patients with seasonal allergic rhinitis. Am Rev Respir Dis 1982;126(4): 625–8.

6. Stuck BA, Czajkowski J, Hagner AE, et al. Changes in daytime sleepiness, quality of life, and objective sleep patterns in seasonal allergic rhinitis: a controlled clinical trial. J Allergy Clin Immunol 2004;113(4):663–8.

7. Young T, Finn L, Kim H. Nasal obstruction as a risk factor for sleep-disordered breathing. The University of Wisconsin Sleep and Respiratory Research Group. J Allergy Clin Immunol 1997;99(2):S757–62.

8. Rundcrantz H. Postural variations of nasal patency. Acta Otolaryngol 1969;68(5):435–43.

9. Kase Y, Hilberg O, Pedersen OF. Posture and nasal patency: evaluation by acoustic rhinometry. Acta Otolaryngol 1994;114(1):70–4.

10. Lal D, Gorges ML, Ungkhara G, et al. Physiological change in nasal patency in response to changes in posture, temperature, and humidity measured by acoustic rhinometry. Am J Rhinol 2006;20(5): 456–62.

11. Virkkula P, Maasilta P, Hytonen M, et al. Nasal obstruction and sleep-disordered breathing: the effect of supine body position on nasal measurements in snorers. Acta Otolaryngol 2003;123(5):648–54.

12. Kiely JL, Nolan P, McNicholas WT. Intranasal corticosteroid therapy for obstructive sleep apnoea in patients with co-existing rhinitis. Thorax 2004;59(1): 50–5.

13. Zwillich CW, Pickett C, Hanson FN, et al. Disturbed sleep and prolonged apnea during nasal obstruction in normal men. Am Rev Respir Dis 1981; 124(2):158–60.

14. Lavie P, Fischel N, Zomer J, et al. The effects of partial and complete mechanical occlusion of the nasal passages on sleep structure and breathing in sleep. Acta Otolaryngol 1983;95(1–2):161–6.

15. Suratt PM, Turner BL, Wilhoit SC. Effect of intranasal obstruction on breathing during sleep. Chest 1986; 90(3):324–9.

16. Tankere F, Maisonobe T, Naccache L, et al. Further evidence for a central reorganisation of synaptic connectivity in patients with hypoglossal-facial anastomosis in man. Brain Res 2000;864(1):87–94.

17. Carberry JC, Hensen H, Fisher LP, et al. Mechanisms contributing to the response of upper-airway muscles to changes in airway pressure. J Appl Physiol (1985) 2015;118(10):1221–8.

18. Lo YL, Jordan AS, Malhotra A, et al. Influence of wakefulness on pharyngeal airway muscle activity. Thorax 2007;62(9):799–805.

19. Wallois F, Macron JM, Jounieaux V, et al. Trigeminal nasal receptors related to respiration and to various stimuli in cats. Respir Physiol 1991;85(1):111–25.

20. Clarke RW, Jones AS. Nasal airflow receptors: the relative importance of temperature and tactile stimulation. Clin Otolaryngol Allied Sci 1992;17(5): 388–92.

21. Aldren C, Tolley NS. Further studies on nasal sensation of airflow. Rhinology 1991;29(1):49–55.

22. White DP, Cadieux RJ, Lombard RM, et al. The effects of nasal anesthesia on breathing during sleep. Am Rev Respir Dis 1985;132(5):972–5.

23. Jordan AS, Wellman A, Heinzer RC, et al. Mechanisms used to restore ventilation after partial upper airway collapse during sleep in humans. Thorax 2007;62(10):861–7.

24. Susarla SM, Thomas RJ, Abramson ZR, et al. Biomechanics of the upper airway: changing concepts in the pathogenesis of obstructive sleep apnea. Int J Oral Maxillofac Surg 2010;39(12): 1149–59.

25. Koutsourelakis I, Georgoulopoulos G, Perraki E, et al. Randomised trial of nasal surgery for fixed nasal obstruction in obstructive sleep apnoea. Eur Respir J 2008;31:110–7.

26. Smith I, Lasserson T, Wright J. Drug therapy for obstructive sleep apnoea in adults. Cochrane Database Syst Rev 2006;(2):CD003002.

27. Clarenbach CF, Kohler M, Senn O, et al. Does nasal decongestion improve obstructive sleep apnea? J Sleep Res 2008;17:444–9.

28. Craig TJ, Mend C, Hughes K, et al. The effect of topical nasal fluticasone on objective sleep testing and the symptoms of rhinitis, sleep, and daytime somnolence in perennial allergic rhinitis. Allergy Asthma Proc 2003;24:53–8.

29. Bahammam AS, Tate R, Manfreda J, et al. Upper airway resistance syndrome: effect of nasal dilation, sleep stage, and sleep position. Sleep 1999;22(5): 592–8.

30. Pevernagie D, Hamans E, Van Cauwenberge P, et al. External nasal dilation reduces snoring in chronic rhinitis patients: a randomized controlled trial. Eur Respir J 2000;15:996–1000.

31. Djupesland PG, Skatvedt O, Borgersen AK. Dichotomous, physiological effects of nocturnal external nasal dilation in heavy snorers: the answer to a rhinologic controversy? Am J Rhinol 2001;15(6): 95–103.

32. Schönhofer B, Kerl J, Suchi S, et al. Effect of nasal valve dilation on effective CPAP level in obstructive sleep apnea. Respir Med 2003;97:1001–5.

33. Scharf MB, McDannold MD, Zaretsky NT, et al. Cyclic alternating pattern sequences in non-apneic snorers with and without nasal dilation. Ear Nose Throat J 1996;75(9):617–9.

34. Ishii L, Roxbury C, Godoy A, et al. Does nasal surgery improve OSA in patients with nasal obstruction and OSA? A meta-analysis. Otolaryngol Head Neck Surg 2015;153:326–33.

35. Li HY, Wang PC, Chen YP, et al. Critical appraisal and meta-analysis of nasal surgery for obstructive sleep apnea. Am J Rhinol Allergy 2011;25(1):45–9.

36. Morinaga M, Nakata S, Yasuma F, et al. Pharyngeal morphology: a determinant of successful nasal surgery for sleep apnea. Laryngoscope 2009;119(5): 1011–6.

37. Li HY, Lee LA, Wang PC, et al. Can nasal surgery improve obstructive sleep apnea: subjective or objective? Am J Rhinol Allergy 2009;23(6):e51–5.

38. Tosun F, Kemikli K, Yetkin S, et al. Impact of endoscopic sinus surgery on sleep quality in patients with chronic nasal obstruction due to nasal polyposis. J Craniofac Surg 2009;20(2):446–9.

39. Li HY, Lin Y, Chen NH, et al. Improvement in quality of life after nasal surgery alone for patients with obstructive sleep apnea and nasal obstruction. Arch Otolaryngol Head Neck Surg 2008;134(4): 429–33.

40. Nakata S, Noda A, Yasuma F, et al. Effects of nasal surgery on sleep quality in obstructive sleep apnea syndrome with nasal obstruction. Am J Rhinol Allergy 2008;22:59–63.

41. Li HY, Lee LA, Wang PC, et al. Nasal surgery for snoring in patients with obstructive sleep apnea. Laryngoscope 2008;118:354–9.

42. Virkkula P, Hytönen M, Bachour A, et al. Smoking and improvement after nasal surgery in snoring men. Am J Rhinol Allergy 2007;21:169–73.

43. Virkkula P, Bachour A, Hytönen M, et al. Snoring is not relieved by nasal surgery despite improvement in nasal resistance. Chest 2006;129(1):81–7.

44. Nakata S, Noda A, Yagi H, et al. Nasal resistance for determinant factor of nasal surgery in CPAP failure patients with obstructive sleep apnea syndrome. Rhinology 2005;43:296–9.

45. Kim ST, Choi JH, Jeon HG, et al. Polysomnographic effects of nasal surgery for snoring and obstructive sleep apnea. Acta Otolaryngol 2004;124:297–300.

46. Verse T, Maurer JT, Pirsig W. Effect of nasal surgery on sleep-related breathing disorders. Laryngoscope 2002;112:64–8.

47. Friedman M, Tanyeri H, Lim JW, et al. Effect of improved nasal breathing on obstructive sleep apnea. Otolaryngol Head Neck Surg 2000;122:71–4.

48. Wu J, Zhao G, Li Y, et al. Apnea-hypopnea index decreased significantly after nasal surgery for obstructive sleep apnea: a meta-analysis. Medicine (Baltimore) 2017;96(5):e6008.

49. Xiao Y, Han D, Zang H, et al. The effectiveness of nasal surgery on psychological symptoms in patients with obstructive sleep apnea and nasal obstruction. Acta Otolaryngol 2016;136:626–32.

50. Shuaib SW, Undavia S, Lin J, et al. Can functional septorhinoplasty independently treat obstructive sleep apnea? Plast Reconstr Surg 2015;135: 1554–65.

51. Yalamanchali S, Cipta S, Waxman J, et al. Effects of endoscopic sinus surgery and nasal surgery in patients with obstructive sleep apnea. Otolaryngol Head Neck Surg 2014;151:171–5.

52. Park CY, Hong JH, Lee JH, et al. Clinical effect of surgical correction for nasal pathology on the treatment of obstructive sleep apnea syndrome. PLoS One 2014;9:e98765.

53. Terzano MG, Parrino L, Sherieri A, et al. Atlas, rules, and recording techniques for the scoring of cyclic alternating pattern (CAP) in human sleep. Sleep Med 2001;2(6):537–53.

54. Weaver TE, Grunstein RR. Adherence to continuous positive airway pressure therapy: the challenge to effective treatment. Proc Am Thorac Soci 2008;5: 173–8.

55. Hoffstein V, Viner S, Mateika S, et al. Treatment of obstructive sleep apnea with nasal continuous positive airway pressure. Patient compliance, perception of benefits, and side effects. Am Rev Respir Dis 1992;145:841–5.

56. Brander PE, Soirinsuo M, Lohela P. Nasopharyngeal symptoms in patients with obstructive sleep apnea syndrome. Effect of nasal CPAP treatment. Respiration 1999;66:128–35.

57. Pepin JL, Leger P, Veale D, et al. Side effects of nasal continuous positive airway pressure in sleep apnea syndrome. Study of 193 patients in two French sleep centers. Chest 1995;107:375–81.

58. Chai-Coetzer CL, Luo YM, Antic NA, et al. Predictors of long-term adherence to continuous positive airway pressure therapy in patients with obstructive sleep apnea and cardiovascular disease in the SAVE study. Sleep 2013;36(12):1929–37.

59. Tagaya M, Otake H, Suzuki K, et al. The comparison of nasal surgery and CPAP on daytime sleepiness in patients with OSAS. Rhinology 2017;55(3): 269–73.

60. Epstein LJ, Kristo D, Strollo PJ Jr, et al, Adult Obstructive Sleep Apnea Task Force of the American Academy of Sleep Medicine. Clinical guideline for the evaluation, management and long-term care of obstructive sleep apnea in adults. J Clin Sleep Med 2009;5(3):263–76.

61. Greiner AN, Hellings PW, Rotiroti G, et al. Allergic rhinitis. Lancet 2011;378:2112–22.

62. Salo PM, Calatroni A, Gergen PJ, et al. Allergy-related outcomes in relation to serum IgE: results from the National Health and Nutrition Examination

Survey 2005–2006. J Allergy Clin Immunol 2011; 127:1226–35.

63. Mims JW. Epidemiology of allergic rhinitis. Int Forum Allergy Rhinol 2014;4(Suppl 2):S18–20.

64. Storms W. Allergic rhinitis-induced nasal congestion: its impact on sleep quality. Prim Care Respir J 2008;17:7–18.

65. Thompson A, Sardana N, Craig TJ. Sleep impairment and daytime sleepiness in patients with allergic rhinitis: the role of congestion and inflammation. Ann Allergy Asthma Immunol 2013;111:446–51.

66. Lofaso F, Coste A, d'Ortho MP, et al. Nasal obstruction as a risk factor for sleep apnoea syndrome. Eur Respir J 2000;16:639–43.

67. Krouse HJ, Davis JE, Krouse JH. Immune mediators in allergic rhinitis and sleep. Otolaryngol Head Neck Surg 2002;126:607–13.

68. Tashiro M, Mochizuki H, Iwabuchi K, et al. Roles of histamine in regulation of arousal and cognition: functional neuroimaging of histamine H1 receptors in human brain. Life Sci 2002;72:409–614.

69. Roxbury CR, Qiu M, Shargorodsky J, et al. Association between allergic rhinitis and poor sleep parameters in U.S. adults. Int Forum Allergy Rhinol 2018; 8(10):1098–106.

70. Lavie P, Gerther R, Zomer J, et al. Breathing disorders in sleep associated with "microarousals" in patients with allergic rhinitis. Acta Otolaryngol 1981;92: 529–33.

71. Young T, Finn L, Palta M. Chronic nasal congestion at night is a risk factor for snoring in a population-based cohort study. Arch Intern Med 2001;161: 1514–9.

72. Udaka T, Suzuki H, Fujimura T, et al. Chronic nasal obstruction causes daytime sleepiness and decreased quality of life even in the absence of snoring. Am J Rhinol 2007;21(5):564–9.

73. Hiraki N, Suzuki H, Shiomori T. Snoring, daytime sleepiness, and nasal obstruction with or without allergic rhinitis. Arch Otolaryngol Head Neck Surg 2008;134(12):1254–7.

Palatal Surgery for Obstructive Sleep Apnea
From Ablation to Reconstruction

Hsueh-Yu Li, MD

KEYWORDS

- Palatal surgery • Uvulopalatopharyngoplasty • Snoring • Obstructive sleep apnea
- Suspension palatoplasty • Relocation pharyngoplasty

KEY POINTS

- Palatal surgery is the paragon among various sleep surgeries since it was the first specially designed surgery and remains widely used surgery for OSA.
- Past history of palatal surgery showed the origin from uvulopalatopharyngoplasty, to mini-invasive sleep surgery, and updated in functional reconstruction on lateral pharyngeal wall and soft palate.
- Palatal reconstruction by hybrid procedure includes excision of tonsils, ablation of adipose tissue and suspension of muscle.
- The integrated treatment of palatal surgery includes reconstruction of airway, restoration of airflow and re-rehabilitation of muscle.

Obstructive sleep apnea (OSA) is a chronic and age-related disease.[1] OSA can be treated with nonsurgical and surgical management of the airway.[2,3] Continuous positive airway pressure (CPAP) is the first-line and gold standard for OSA.[2] Acceptance of the device, compliance rate, and long-term adherence, however, are obstacles for its wide use in OSA patients. Poor compliance of CPAP commonly exists in young and mild OSA patients without daytime sleepiness.[4] Surgery is an alternative and salvage treatment to those patients who are unwilling or intolerant to CPAP therapy. Among various sleep surgeries, palatal surgery was the first surgical procedure specifically designed to treat snoring and OSA.[3] Traditional palatal surgery in terms of uvulopalatopharyngoplasty (UPPP) includes removal of the tonsils and excision of the redundant pillars, soft palate, and uvula.[3] Although UPPP alleviates clinical symptoms of OSA, it was criticized for severe postoperative pain, related complications, and low success rate.[5] In the past few decades, palatal surgery with many modifications remains the most commonly used operation for snoring and OSA. In this article, the history of palatal surgery is introduced to have a further understanding of its evolution from past procedures to future development. Furthermore, changes of palatal surgery for OSA are discussed in surgical indication (what is the purpose), obstruction site (how to diagnosis), and treatment endpoint (when to stop). Moreover, the hybrid palatal technique is presented form ablation to reconstruction. Finally, palatal surgery is in conjunction with postoperative myofunctional therapy (MFT) to fulfill the integrated treatment of OSA.

HISTORICAL EVOLUTION OF PALATAL SURGERY FOR OBSTRUCTIVE SLEEP APNEA

In the 1950s, resection of soft palate triangles paramedian to the uvula has been implemented in surgical procedure for snoring (**Table 1**).[6,7] This technique enhanced the relationship between

Department of Otolaryngology, Chang Gung Memorial Hospital, 333, No 5, Fushing Street, Gueishan Shiang, Taoyuan, Taiwan
E-mail address: hyli38@cgmh.org.tw

Sleep Med Clin 14 (2019) 51–58
https://doi.org/10.1016/j.jsmc.2018.10.006
1556-407X/19/© 2018 Elsevier Inc. All rights reserved.

Table 1
Historical evolution of palatal surgery for obstructive sleep apnea

Year/Concept	Procedure
1950	Resection of soft palate triangle
1960	Amputation of the uvula
1970	Tracheostomy
1980	UPPP
1990	LAUP
Ablation	RF ablation
2000	Pillar implant
Reconstruction	Lateral palatoplasty Expansion sphincter pharyngoplasty Z-palatoplasty Relocation pharyngoplasty
2010	Barbed reposition pharyngoplasty Suspension palatoplasty

velum and snoring, and inspired the following palatal surgery.

In the 1960s, amputation of the uvula (uvulectomy) was initiated to ameliorate snoring with more changes in pitch from reduction in the amplitude of vibration.[8]

In the 1970s, tracheostomy via permanent stoma was the model treatment of pickwickian syndrome and OSA with severe daytime sleepiness.[9] Related comorbidities and the development of CPAP, however, prohibit its clinical use.

In the 1980s, the introduction of UPPP by Fujita and colleagues[3] was the contemporary surgical milestone in treating snoring and OSA. UPPP enlarged and stabilized the oropharyngeal airway and consequently decrease airway collapse and airflow turbulence. Simmons[10] advocated removing the soft palate as much as possible and became a general impression of UPPP (classic UPPP). General outcomes of UPPP revealed significant improvement of subjective symptoms in conjunction with incongruous changes in polysomnography.

Striding forward to 1990s, laser-assisted uvulopalatoplasty (LAUP) using a CO_2 laser to vaporize the vibrating uvula and soft palate launched a series of office-based antisnore procedures.[11] Although LAUP improves habitual snoring, the scarring effect can narrow the velopharyngeal airway and exacerbate OSA. In the late 1990s, radiofrequency (RF) was introduced as interstitial thermotherapy. RF to the soft palate is mini-invasive without major complications.[12] The antisnore effect of RF, however, declines sharply with time and commonly requires repeated sessions to achieve optimal results.[13]

In the early 2000s, pillar implant, acting as an extension of the hard palate, was introduced to stiffen the broad and long soft palate in a single application.[14] Pillar implant improved snoring in primary snorers and needs combination with other treatment modalities in more severe and intense SRBD.[15] At the same time, many modifications of UPPP technique were implemented, trying to stabilize the lateral pharyngeal wall and prevent its collapse to improve sleep apnea.[16–19]

In 2010s, there was an increased interest in suspending palatopharyngeus muscle to the pterygomandibular raphe for further enlargement of the velopharyngeal airspace.[20,21]

CONCEPTUAL EVOLUTION OF PALATAL SURGERY

Changes of palatal surgery for OSA in thought include the surgical indication (what is the purpose), obstruction site (how to diagnosis), and treatment endpoint (when to stop).

Surgical Purpose

OSA is a chronic disease, like hypertension, diabetes, and asthma, and surgery is more likely to improve instead of cure the disease. Evidence shows that palatal surgery significantly alleviates OSA-related symptoms and reduces the risk of major complications but rarely normalizes apnea/hypopnea index (AHI).[5,22–24] Furthermore, recent evidence shows that OSA patients have higher prevalence in vertigo, tinnitus, and sudden deafness than the matched non-OSA population, which may be attributable to hypoxemia to the inner ear.[25–27] Further reports showed that the use of CPAP improved inner ear symptoms in OSA patients.[27,28] Consequently, vertigo, tinnitus, and sudden deafness are likely to be additional indications for surgical OSA patients.

Obstruction Site

Traditional assessment of airway obstruction for palatal surgery in treating OSA includes physical examination (Friedman stage), nasopharyngoscopy with Müller maneuver, and lateral cephalometry. They are all implemented in wakefulness and inconsistent with those detected during sleep, particularly at the hypopharyngeal and laryngeal obstruction.[29] Therefore, drug-induced sleep endoscopy (DISE) becomes a prerequisite for decision making of the surgical plan for OSA patients.[30] The advantage of DISE is to provide simulate dynamic airway collapse during pharmacologically induced sleep. Reports revealed that complete concentric collapse at the velopharynx was associated with higher body mass index and surgical failure.[29,31] Advancement in drug-induced sleep imaging can offer dynamic airway movement in a sagittal view that can demonstrate uvular/velar collapse and the interaction of palate/tongue collapse for decision making of surgical plan.[32]

Endpoint

Postoperative AHI is used to classify surgical success or failure of OSA. OSA, however, is a chronic and presumably lifelong disease that makes it unrealistic to cure. Therefore, normalization of AHI is not an endpoint for OSA. Furthermore, research has revealed that change of AHI is not consistent with improvement of clinical symptoms (a major concern for patients). Improvement in either AHI or clinical symptoms is incomplete. The real goal in treating OSA should be to improve the disease in terms of AHI reduction and ameliorate symptoms and minimize ongoing sequence. Therefore, the endpoint of palatal surgery for OSA is suggested as follows: (1) significant improvement of major complaints, (2) postoperative AHI less than 15/h, and (3) low risk in biomarkers of coronary artery/cardiovascular disease.[4]

TECHNIQUE EVOLUTION—FROM ABLATION TO RECONSTRUCTION

Palatal surgery plays a key role in intrapharyngeal surgery (soft tissue–targeted surgery) for OSA. There is no widely accepted guideline or algorithm in patient selection for palatal surgery. Based on individual training background and facility possessed, surgeons use their judgment for patient selection. Preoperative airway assessment, however, is a prerequisite for patient selection and airway anatomy–based staging is more reliable than disease severity–based staging in the outcomes of palatal surgery for OSA.[33] Several anatomic factors may contribute to a good surgical outcome of palatal surgery large tonsils, including elongated uvula, pliable posterior pillars (webbing), low Friedman tongue position, absence of macroglossia in the oropharyngeal examination, nonconcentric collapse of the velopharynx, absence of tongue and epiglottis collapse in DISE, thin and long soft palate without craniofacial anomaly in lateral cephalometry, and absence of morbid obesity in physical examination.[34] Based on these criteria, only one-fourth of OSA patients were considered good candidates with favorable anatomy for palatal surgery.[34] These findings enhance the fact that a vast majority of OSA patients have multilevel

obstruction and explains the suboptimal outcomes of palatal surgery despite technical endeavor. Therefore, palatal surgery is usually applied as part of multilevel surgery for OSA in surgical algorithm. Combined nasal and palatal surgery is more commonly used than simultaneous palatal and hypopharyngeous surgery.[35–37]

Palatal surgery for OSA is still in evolutionary change. UPPP includes 2 parts palatoplasty for soft palate collapse and pharyngoplasty for lateral pharyngeal wall collapse (**Fig. 1**). Classical excision of redundant soft palate incurred severe postoperative pain and velopharyngeal insufficiency that further jeopardized salvage use of CPAP in surgical failure patients because of mouth leak.[10,38] Accordingly, evolving procedures of palatal surgery are removing tissue from the lateral pharyngeal wall and conservative resection of the palate and uvula.[16–19] Ablation techniques, although mini-invasive, generally result in limited effect that commonly declines sharply with time and needs repeated sessions.[39] To minimize the side effect and maximize the surgical efficacy, palatal surgery for OSA is changing from radical excision of the soft palate, mini-invasive ablation toward a hybrid model reconstruction. Hybrid model reconstruction in the palatal surgery can be classified as histologic gradation: (1) mucosa: preservation; (2) adipose tissue: ablation; (3) muscle: suspension; and (4) lymphoid tissue: excision (**Fig. 2**).

Preservation of the mucosa (see **Fig. 2**) is important in the reduction of suture tension to decrease wound dehiscence and lessen postoperative pain,

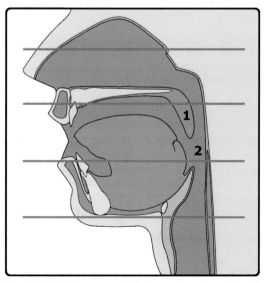

Fig. 1. Palatal surgery includes palatoplasty for (1) soft palate collapse and pharyngoplasty for (2) lateral pharyngeal wall collapse.

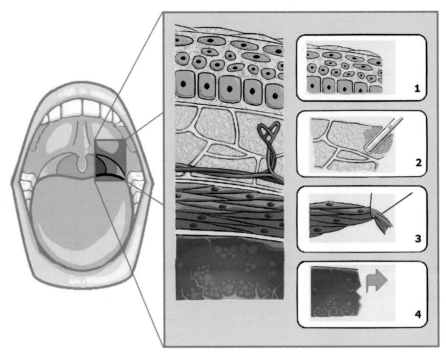

Fig. 2. Hybrid reconstruction of the palatal surgery can be classified into histologic gradation: (1) mucosa: preservation; (2) adipose tissue: ablation; (3) muscle: suspension; and (4) lymphoid tissue: excision.

in maintenance of submucosal gland secretion to ameliorate dryness of the mouth, and to curtail raw wound to facilitate wound healing.

Accumulation of palatal adipose tissue can thicken the soft palate, narrow the velopharyngeal airspace, and cause velopharyngeal obstruction. With the development of ablation procedures, reduction of palatal fat can be achieved via a mini-invasive approach with similar effect (see **Fig. 2**). Palatal ablation through upper pole of tonsillar fossa after tonsillectomy (intrawound approach) is a mode without additional damage of palatal mucosa.

Suspension of pharyngeal muscle is key in the hybrid reconstruction of palatal surgery (see **Fig. 2**). Suspension instead of excision of pharyngeal muscle in palatal surgery for OSA augments the pharyngeal airway to improve respiration, moreover, with no damage to normal pharyngeal function in terms of phonation and swallowing.

Lymphoid tissue (palatal tonsil) is the only tissue to be excised in the hybrid reconstruction of palatal surgery (see **Fig. 2**). Tonsillectomy is mandatory to widen the oropharyngeal air lumen and facilitate reconstruction of lateral pharyngeal wall.

Velopharyngeal obstruction can be divided into lateral, anterior-posterior (A-P), and concentric collapse under observation during DISE in VOTE classification.[30]

Lateral pharyngeal wall collapse was deemed a determinant factor in contributing to OSA.[40] Image study showed progressive narrowing or expanding in the lateral dimension of the upper airway on continuous negative pressure or continuous positive pressure implemented.[41] The use of suspension maneuver for lateral pharyngeal wall collapse has been implemented in individual techniques.[16,17,19] Lateral pharyngoplasty was used to ameliorate lateral pharyngeal wall collapse by suturing the lateral flap of superior pharyngeal constrictor muscle to the palatoglossus muscle.[16] Expansion sphincter pharyngoplasty isolated and rotated the palatopharyngeus muscle superoanterolaterally to create the lateral pharyngeal wall tension.[17] Relocation pharyngoplasty reconstructed the tonsillar fossa by splinting the medial flap of superior pharyngeal constrictor muscle to the palatoglossus muscle.[19] Barbed reposition pharyngoplasty uses a knotless bidirectional reabsorbable stitch to outer mucosal suture the palatopharyngeus muscle with pterygomandibular raphe.[20]

A-P collapse of the soft palate is another type of velopharyngeal obstruction. It exists commonly in less obese patients with small tonsils.[21] Traditional UPPP showed no benefit in these OSA patients. Suspension palatoplasty identifies the pterygomandibular raphe and suspends the palatopharyngeus muscle to the raphe in A-P collapse of the velopharynx (**Fig. 3**).[21] **Fig. 4** demonstrates

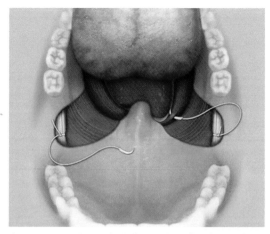

Fig. 3. Suspension palatoplasty identifies the pterygomandibular raphe and suspends the palatopharyngeus muscle to the raphe.

the perioperative changes in retropalatal space (70° rigid endoscopy, transnasal) and posterior air space (lateral cephalometry) in 1 patient.

For concentric collapse, a combined A-P and lateral suspension is needed for comprehensive improvement of the collapse from all directions.

Previous studies showed no velopharyngeal insufficiency in terms of changes in voice, articulation, and nasality after relocation pharyngoplasty.[42] The authors presume those surgeries not only advance but also elevate soft palate, facilitating the contraction of the levator veli palatini muscle to separate the nasopharynx and oropharynx during swallowing and phonation.[42] Surgical results are superior to traditional UPPP in the reduction of sleep apnea.[16–21]

Some specific palatal surgical techniques are used in specific condition of velopharyngeal obstruction. Zetapalatopharyngoplasty splits the uvula and soft palate in the midline and reflects the palatal flaps laterally to widen the retropalatal space particularly in previous tonsillectomy patients.[18] Transpalatal advancement pharyngoplasty excises the hard palate and advances the palatal flap to pull forward and superior the palate similar to maxillary advancement.[43] Extended uvulopalatal flap removed the anterior palatal adipose tissue and relocates the soft palate anterior and lateral and is implemented more than in thick (>1.5 cm) soft palate.[44] Septal cartilage implant is an alternative to pillar implant in strengthening the collapsible soft palate with the advantage in tailor-made implants for individual lengths of soft palate.[45]

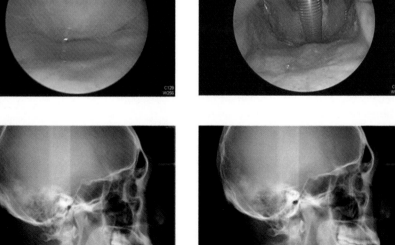

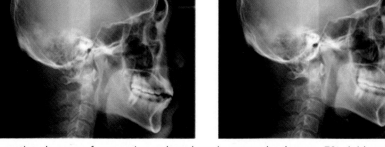

Fig. 4. Perioperative changes of suspension palatoplasty in retropalatal space, 70° rigid endoscopy (transnasal: [*upper left*] preoperative and [*upper right*] postoperative) and posterior air space (lateral cephalometry: [*lower left*] preoperative and [*lower left*] postoperative) in 1 patient.

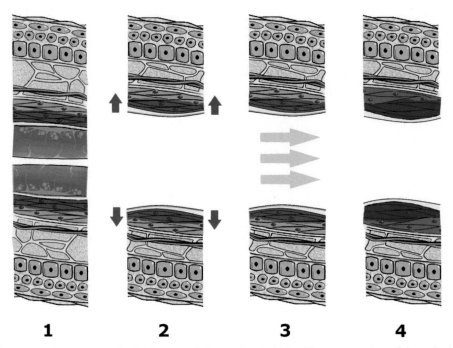

Fig. 5. (1) Integrated treatment of velopharyngeal obstruction includes (2) reconstruction of the velopharyngeal airway, (3) restoration of the velopharyngeal airflow, and (4) re-education of the oropharyngeal muscle.

POSTOPERATIVE EVOLUTION—FROM HOSPITAL WOUND CARE TO HOME MUSCLE EDUCATION

OSA patients who have undergone palatal surgery are usually hospitalized 1 day to 2 days, and the hospitalization period can be longer if multilevel surgery is performed.

Postoperative hospital care involves humidified oxygen support (CPAP can be an alternative to oxygen supply if the patient is a CPAP user), positional therapy, prophylactic antibiotic, pain control by intravenous ketoprofen (Ketololac) (intravenous cyclooxygenase 2 for nonsteroidal anti-inflammatory drug allergy), topical anesthetics (benzocaine or Difflam), corticosteroid ointment (Kenalog) application, and ice packing on submental area.

The criteria for discharge are stable vital signs, adequate pain control, oral intake of soft diet, and good healing of wound without bleeding.

After complete healing of the wound, palatal surgery significantly improves snoring, daytime sleepiness, and quality of life in short-term follow up. The outcomes of palatal surgery, however, usually decline with time because of maturity of operation scar and weakening of muscle tone in aging. Therefore, there is a necessity of oropharyngeal MFT as conjunctive treatment to re-educate the oropharyngeal muscles to enhance and sustain the surgical outcomes. Accordingly, the management of velopharyngeal obstruction can proceed from baseline obstruction, reconstruction of the velopharyngeal airway, restoration of the velopharyngeal airflow, to re-education of the oropharyngeal muscle (**Fig. 5**).

MFT includes oropharyngeal muscle exercise and posture and respiration training.[46] MFT is best implemented in middle-aged, nonobese, mild/moderate OSA patients.[47] The muscles of the soft palate, tongue, lateral pharyngeal wall, temporo-mastoid joint, face and neck are exercised and trained.[48] MFT is composed of mode (isotonic/isometric), intensity (progressive usually), frequency (2–3/wk commonly), and duration (3 months/course generally) that can be personalized in individual patients.[49] Studies showed oropharyngeal exercises improved sleep apnea and neck circumference in patients with moderate OSA.[49] Clinical application of MFT as conjunctive treatment after palatal surgery revealed the improvement of snoring intensity, lumping, tight sensation of the throat, drooling, and mouth breathing.

SUMMARY

The management of velopharyngeal obstruction by palatal surgery is a key treatment in OSA patients. The evolution of palatal surgery changes is from radical excision, to mini-invasive ablation, toward hybrid model reconstruction of the velopharynx. Suspension of pharyngeal muscle is the core value in the widening of the airway. Postoperative MFT is important to enhance and maintain surgical outcomes.

ACKNOWLEDGMENTS

The author would like to express deepest gratitude to Linkou-Chang Gung Memorial Hospital for long term support by grants in our sleep research and thank Mr. Cheng-Shian Tsai for the illustrations.

REFERENCES

1. Young T, Palta M, Dempsey J, et al. The occurrence of sleep-disordered breathing among middle-aged adults. N Engl J Med 1993;328:1230–5.
2. Sullivan CE, Issa FG, Berthon-Jones M, et al. Reversal of obstructive sleep apnoea by continuous positive airway pressure applied through the nares. Lancet 1981;1(8225):862–5.
3. Fujita S, Conway W, Zorick F, et al. Surgical correction of anatomic abnormalities in obstructive sleep apnea syndrome: uvulopalatopharyngoplasty. Otolaryngol Head Neck Surg 1981;89:923–34.
4. Li HY. Updated palate surgery for obstructive sleep apnea. In: Lin HC, editor. Sleep-related breathing disorders. Adv otorhinolaryngol, vol. 80. Basel (Switzerland): Karger; 2017. p. 74–80.
5. Sher AE, Schechtman KB, Piccirrillo JF. The efficacy of surgical modifications of the upper airway in adults with obstructive sleep apnea syndrome. Sleep 1996;19:156–77.
6. Yaremchuk K, Garcia-Rodriguez L. The history of sleep surgery. In: Lin HC, editor. Sleep-related breathing disorders. Adv otorhinolaryngol, vol. 80. Basel (Switzerland): Karger; 2017. p. 74–80.
7. Heinberg CJ. A surgical procedure for the relief of snoring. Eye Ear Nose Throat Mon 1955;34:389.
8. Robin I. Snoring. (abridged version). Proc R Soc Med 1968;61:575–82.
9. Weitzman ED, Pollack CP, Borowiecki B. Hypersomnia-sleep apnea due to micrognathia: reversal by tracheoplasty. Arch Neurol 1978;35:392–5.
10. Simmons FB, Guilleminault C, Silvestri R. Snoring and some obstructive sleep apnea can be cured by oropharyngeal surgery. Arch Otolaryngol 1983;109:503–7.
11. Kamami Y. Laser CO2 for snoring, preliminary results. Acta Otorhinolaryngol Belg 1990;44:45–6.
12. Powell NB, Riley RW, Troell RJ, et al. Radiofrequency volumetric tissue reduction of the palate in subjects with sleep-disordered breathing. Chest 1998;113:1163–74.
13. Li KK, Powell NB, Riley RW, et al. Radiofrequency volumetric reduction of the palate: an extended follow-up study. Otolaryngol Head Neck Surg 2000;122:410–4.
14. Ho WK, Wei WI, Chung KF. Managing disturbing snoring with palatal implants: a pilot study. Arch Otolaryngol Head Neck Surg 2004;130:753–8.
15. Friedman M, Vidyasagar R, Bliznikas D, et al. Patient selection and efficacy of Pillar implant technique for treatment of snoring and obstructive sleep apnea/hypopnea syndrome. Otolaryngol Head Neck Surg 2006;134:187–96.
16. Cahali MB. Lateral pharyngoplasty: a new treatment for obstructive sleep apneahypopnea syndrome. Laryngoscope 2003;113:1961–8.
17. Pang KP, Woodson BT. Expansion sphincter pharyngoplasty: a new technique for the treatment of obstructive sleep apnea. Otolaryngol Head Neck Surg 2007;137:110–4.
18. Friedman M, Ibrahim HZ, Vidyasagar R, et al. Z-palatoplasty (ZPP): a technique for patients without tonsils. Otolaryngol Head Neck Surg 2004;131:89–100.
19. Li HY, Lee LA. Relocation pharyngoplasty for obstructive sleep apnea. Laryngoscope 2009;119:2472–7.
20. Vicini C, Hendawy E, Campanini A, et al. Barbed reposition pharyngoplasty (BRP) for OSAHS: a feasibility, safety, efficacy and teachability pilot study. "We are on the giant's shoulder". Eur Arch Otorhinolaryngol 2015;272:3065–70.
21. Li HY, Lee LA, Kezirian EJ, et al. Suspension palatoplasty for obstructive sleep apnea- a preliminary study. Sci Rep 2018. https://doi.org/10.1038/s41598-018-22710-1.
22. Li HY, Chen NH, Shu YH, et al. Changes of quality of life and respiratory disturbance after extended uvulopalatal flap surgery in patients with obstructive sleep apnea. Arch Otolaryngol Head Neck Surg 2004;130:195–200.
23. Li HY, Huang YS, Chen NH, et al. Mood improvement after surgery for obstructive sleep apnea. Laryngoscope 2004;116:1098–102.
24. Li HY, Lee LA, Yu JF, et al. Changes of snoring sound after relocation pharyngoplasty for obstructive sleep apnoea: the surgery reduces mean intensity in snoring which correlates well to apnoea-hypopnoea index. Clin Otolaryngol 2015;40:98–105.
25. Tsai MS, Lee LA, Tsai YT, et al. Sleep apnea and risk of vertigo: a nationwide population-based cohort study. Laryngoscope 2018;128:763–8.
26. Sheu JJ, Wu CS, Lin HC. Association between obstructive sleep apnea and sudden sensorineural hearing loss. Arch Otolaryngol Head Neck Surg 2012;138:55–9.
27. Lai JT, Shen PH, Lin CY, et al. Higher prevalence and increased severity of sleep-disordered breathing in

male patients with chronic tinnitus: our experience with 173 cases. Clin Otolaryngol 2018;43:722–5.

28. Nakayama M. A pilot study on the efficacy of continuous positive airway pressure on the manifestations of Ménière's disease in patients with concomitant obstructive sleep apnea syndrome. J Clin Sleep Med 2015;11:1101–10.

29. Certal VF, Pratas R, Guimaraes L, et al. Awake examination versus DISE for surgical decision making in patients with OSA: a systemic review. Laryngoscope 2016;126:768–74.

30. Kezirian EJ, Hohenhorst W, de Vries N. Drug-induced sleep endoscopy: the VOTE classification. Eur Arch Otorhinolaryngol 2011;268:1233–6.

31. Koutsourelakis I, Safiruddin F, Ravesloot M, et al. Surgery for obstructive sleep apnea: sleep endoscopy determinants of outcome. Laryngoscope 2012;122:2587–91.

32. Li HY, Lo YL, Wang CJ, et al. Dynamic drug- induced sleep computed tomography in adults with obstructive sleep apnea. Sci Rep 2016;6:35849.

33. Li HY, Wang PC, Li LA, et al. Prediction of uvulopalatopharyngoplasty outcome: anatomy-based staging system versus severity-based staging system. Sleep 2006;29:1537–41.

34. Katsantonis GP. Uvulopalatopharyngoplasty. Sleep apnea and snoring-surgical and non-surgical therapy. In: Friedman M, editorvol. 29. Saunders, Elsevier; 2009. p. 176–83.

35. Li HY, Wang PC, Hsu CY, et al. Concomitant nasal and palatopharyngeal surgery for obstructive sleep apnea: simultaneous or staged. Acta Otolaryngol 2005;125:298–303.

36. Li HY, Wang PC, Hsu CY, et al. Same-stage palatopharyngeal and hypopharyngeal surgery for severe obstructive sleep apnea. Acta Otolaryngol 2004; 124:820–6.

37. Kezirian EJ, Goldberg AN. Hypopharyngeal surgery in obstructive sleep apnea. Arch Otolaryngol Head Neck Surg 2006;132:206–13.

38. Mortimore IL, Bradley PA, Murray JA, et al. UPPP may compromise nasal CPAP therapy in sleep apnea syndrome. Am J Respir Crit Care Med 1996; 154:1759–62.

39. Veer V, Yang WY, Green R, et al. Long-term safety and efficacy of radiofrequency ablation in the treatment of sleep disordered breathing: a meta-analysis. Eur Arch Otorhinolaryngol 2014;271:2863–70.

40. Schwab RJ, Gupta KB, Gefter WB, et al. Upper airway and soft tissue anatomy in normal subjects and patients with sleep disordered breathing: significance of the lateral pharyngeal walls. Am J Respir Crit Care Med 1995;152:1673–89.

41. Schwab RJ, Gefter WB, Hoffman EA, et al. Dynamic upper airway imaging during awake respiration in normal subjects and patients with sleep disordered breathing. Am Rev Respir Dis 1993;148:1385–400.

42. Li HY, Lee LA, Fang TJ, et al. Evaluation of velopharyngeal function after relocation pharyngoplasty for obstructive sleep apnea. Laryngoscope 2010;120: 1069–73.

43. Woodson BT, Toohill RJ. Transpalatal advancement pharyngoplasty for obstructive sleep apnea. Laryngoscope 1993;103:269–76.

44. Li HY, Li KK, Chen NH, et al. Modified uvulopalatopharyngoplasty: the extended uvulopalatal flap. Am J Otolaryngol 2003;24:311–6.

45. Lee YC, Lee LA, Li HY. The palatal septal cartilage implantation for snoring and obstructive sleep apnea. Auris Nasus Larynx 2018;45:1199–205.

46. Villa MP, Brasili L, Ferretti A, et al. Oropharyngeal exercises to reduce symptoms of OSA after AT. Sleep Breath 2015;19:281–9.

47. Camacho M, Guilleminault C, Wei JM, et al. Oropharyngeal and tongue exercises (myofunctional therapy) for snoring: a systematic review and meta-analysis. Eur Arch Otorhinolaryngol 2018;275: 849–55.

48. Guimarães KC, Drager LF, Genta PR, et al. Effects of oropharyngeal exercises on patients with moderate obstructive sleep apnea syndrome. Am J Respir Crit Care Med 2009;179:962–6.

49. Camacho M, Certal V, Abdullatif J, et al. Myofunctional therapy to treat obstructive sleep apnea: a systematic review and meta-analysis. Sleep 2015; 38:669–75.

Volumetric Tongue Reduction for Obstructive Sleep Apnea

Hsin-Ching Lin, MD[a],*, Michael Friedman, MD[b,c]

KEYWORDS

- Volumetric tongue reduction • Obstructive sleep apnea • Continuous positive airway pressure

KEY POINTS

- The hypopharyngeal/tongue base procedures for the treatment of obstructive sleep apnea/hypopnea syndrome (OSA) are usually challenging to most sleep surgeons.
- In recent years, several procedures for OSA patients with hypopharyngeal obstructions have been developed to achieve higher response rates with decreased postoperative morbidities.
- This article presents an overview and pitfalls of volumetric tongue base resection for the treatment of OSA.

INTRODUCTION

A perusal of the advancements made in obstructive sleep apnea (OSA) surgery shows that hypopharynx/tongue base surgery has remained a challenge for most sleep surgeons. Traditional hypopharyngeal/tongue base procedures for OSA are usually aggressive and technically advanced.[1] Some previously reported cases even needed temporary postoperative tracheotomy. Kezirian and colleagues[2] reported on the types of surgeries performed for OSA in the United States. They found that only 18.6% of the enrolled 35,263 OSA surgeries involved hypopharyngeal surgery. The study investigated practice patterns, perceptions, and attitudes for hypopharyngeal surgery in OSA with a cross-sectional online survey of American Academy of Otolaryngology–Head and Neck Surgery Foundation members via a 5-point Likert scale. The results showed that

more than 40% of respondents reported limited experience on training for individual hypopharyngeal procedures.[3] Furthermore, Brietzke and colleagues[4] reported the national database analysis of single-level versus multilevel sleep surgery in the United States for the years 2010 through 2012. Their study cohort included 14,633 patients and only a total of 12.65% involved the base of the tongue (BOT)/hypopharyngeal OSA surgery (1164 patients [7.95%] underwent uvulopalatopharyngoplasty [UPPP] plus tongue/hypopharyngeal surgery and 691 patients [4.7%] underwent UPPP combined with nasal and tongue/hypopharyngeal surgery).

In 2006, Kezirian and Goldberg[5] performed an evidence-based medicine review of the literature describing outcomes of hypopharyngeal surgery on OSA patients. Their results showed that successful outcomes were achieved in 35% to 62%

Competing Interests: Dr H.-C. Lin received research grants from Intuitive Surgical Inc., Sunnyvale., CA, USA. However, Intuitive Surgical Inc., had no role in the design or conduct of this article. This study was supported by grants CMRPG8F0421 and CMRPG8F0422, Chang Gung Memorial Hospital, Kaohsiung, Taiwan; Intuitive Surgical Inc., Sunnyvale, CA, USA.

[a] Department of Otolaryngology, Sleep Center, Robotic Surgery Center, Kaohsiung Chang Gung Memorial Hospital, 123, Ta-Pei Road, Niao-Sung District, Kaohsiung City 833, Taiwan; [b] Division of Sleep Surgery, Department of Otolaryngology–Head and Neck Surgery, Rush University Medical Center, 1653 West Congress Parkway, Chicago, IL 60612, USA; [c] Department of Otolaryngology, Advanced Center for Specialty Care, Advocate Illinois Masonic Medical Center, 836 West Wellington Avenue, Chicago, IL 60657, USA
* Corresponding author.
E-mail addresses: hclin@adm.cgmh.org.tw; enthclin@aol.com

Sleep Med Clin 14 (2019) 59–65
https://doi.org/10.1016/j.jsmc.2018.10.007

of patients when considering the improvement in respiratory physiology alone and that certain subgroups achieved higher success rates. They concluded that hypopharyngeal surgery in OSA is associated with improved outcomes, although this benefit is supported largely by level 4 evidence.

In 2015, Murphey and colleagues[6] reported the results of an updated systematic review and meta-analysis on the effects of glossectomy as part of multilevel sleep surgery on OSA patients. Their study enrolled a total of 18 articles with 522 patients treated with 3 glossectomy techniques (midline glossectomy, lingualplasty, and submucosal minimally invasive lingual excision). Pooled analyses showed a significant improvement in apnea/hypopnea index (AHI, per hour), Epworth Sleepiness Scale, snoring visual analog scale, and lowest O_2 saturation. Surgical success rate was 59.6% (95% confidence interval [CI], 53.0%-65.9%), and surgical cure was achieved in 22.5% (95% CI, 11.26%-36.26%) of cases. They also concluded that glossectomy significantly improves sleep outcomes as part of multilevel surgery in adult patients with OSA.

Tracheotomy was the first surgical treatment of OSA. It can shunt the entire upper airway and is effective; however, most patients and physicians could not accept it as a permanent form for treating patients with OSA. Traditional tongue-base surgeries, such as transcervical tongue base reduction with hyoepiglottoplasty, midline laser glossectomy, tongue base suspension, genioglossus advancement, and hyoid suspension, are effective only to a certain degree. These traditional procedures are intrusive and often associated with complications, including edema, infection, bleeding, lingual paralysis, and persistent odynophagia.[1,7–11]

In recent years, several procedures for OSA patients with hypopharyngeal obstructions have been developed to achieve higher response rates with decreased postoperative morbidities via the advancement of medical technology. The surgeries of the BOT include both resection and suspension of the tongue tissues. The procedures available to treat tongue/hypopharyngeal obstructions in OSA include genioglossus advancement, mortised genioplasty, tongue radiofrequency treatment, surgical reduction of the tongue base, hyoepiglottoplasty, hyoid suspension, and tongue base stabilization. These procedures can be performed alone or in combination under the same anesthetic course. The following sections discuss the important issues of major procedures on volumetric tongue base reduction for OSA.

INDICATIONS AND CONTRAINDICATION FOR TONGUE BASE OBSTRUCTIVE SLEEP APNEA SURGERY

The indications include the following:

1. Significant symptoms of habitual snoring and/or excessive daytime somnolence,
2. AHI (events/h) greater than 5,
3. Failure or refusal of attempts at conservative treatments, such as oral appliances or continuous positive airway pressure (CPAP) therapy,
4. Friedman tongue position[12,13] III/IV,
5. Retrolingual/hypopharyngeal obstructions identified by the Mueller maneuver on endoscopy and/or propofol-induced sleep endoscopy,
6. Body mass index <40 kg/m^2.
7. Age more than 18 year old is optional.

Contraindications are as follows:

1. Contraindications for general anesthesia,
2. Severe trismus and mouth opening less than 2 fingers' width (~3 cm) may not have adequate space for these procedures,
3. Poor dentition, increasing the difficulty to use the mouth gag retractor,
4. Patients with known severe swallowing or speech problems preoperatively.

Patients should continue to take regularly scheduled medications, especially antihypertensive medicine, up to and including the morning of surgery. Exceptions may include anticoagulants to avoid increased surgical bleeding and oral hypoglycemic drugs. Patients must inform the possibility of postoperative taste disturbance after the procedure, especially in special careers such as chef or sommelier.

RADIOFREQUENCY SURGERY FOR OBSTRUCTIVE SLEEP APNEA

A minimally invasive technique that was first developed for tongue base reduction in patients with retrolingual obstruction is radiofrequency ablation at the tongue base (RFBOT). Radiofrequency application to the field of sleep surgery using the Somnus system was first reported by Powell in 1998.[14] This system principally used a monopolar device, but subsequently many other devices were introduced that used bipolar technology with some acting in wet medium. Such devices include Coblator, Celon, Sutter, and Ellman.[15] The generator of energy delivery is different with each different system used. Some systems allow only interstitial thermotherapy, whereas others offer electrosection in addition to removing some part of the long uvula or redundant webbing at the free edge of the soft palate. Generally, bipolar systems release less power and cause less heat energy dissipation allowing for more accurate thermal energy to be delivered.[15] Stimpson and Kotecha[16] demonstrated the advantage of radiofrequency over laser as a surgical tool at the cellular level.

The success rate has been reported to be between 20% and 83% with RFBOT. The basis of this procedure is volume reduction due to coagulation necrosis and scar contraction. A 17% reduction in the tongue base volume has been shown as a result of a mean of 5.5 applications of RFBOT,[17] but this is still not sufficient for patients with moderate/severe disease requiring relatively aggressive tongue base treatment. Other negative aspects of this technique, along with the insufficient success rate, are the number of applications and the frequency of hospitalizations.

Babademez and colleagues[18] compared the effectiveness and morbidity of 3 microinvasive tongue base surgical procedures (low-temperature bipolar radiofrequency, submucosal minimally invasive lingual excision with radiofrequency, and submucosal minimally invasive lingual excision with a harmonic scalpel) combined with UPPP. They found that UPPP plus submucosal minimally invasive lingual excision with radiofrequency/coblation was found to be more effective when the polysomnography findings were evaluated.

In the authors' study,[19] the SMILE (submucosal minimally invasive lingual excision with coblation) technique for tongue base reduction demonstrated increased efficacy over RFBOT but resulted in more complications in a comparable surgical protocol for OSA. Patients in both groups demonstrated a significant reduction in AHI. Success rates for SMILE and RFBOT were 64.6% and 41.7%, respectively ($P = .024$).

In the authors' practice, patients underwent RFBOT (Somnoplasty System, Gyrus Inc, Memphis, TN, USA) as treatment of the tongue base obstruction. Patients usually received 4500 to 7500 J distributed to 6 to 10 points along the midline of the tongue behind the circumvallate papillae.

ENDOSCOPIC COBLATION TONGUE BASE RESECTION FOR OBSTRUCTIVE SLEEP APNEA

With the use of coblation® technology (plasma-mediated radiofrequency; Smith & Nephew Inc., Andover, MA, USA), which provides relatively low temperature (40°C – 70°C), and thermal injury to the target lesion and surrounding tissues, an alternative approach called SMILE with coblation was developed in an effort to maximize tongue base

reduction using a minimally invasive technique. In 2006, Maturo and Mair[20] reported the anatomic dissection of fresh cadavers and a representative case series of children who underwent SMILE under intraoral ultrasonic and endoscopic guidance. In the authors' prior study,[9] they compared the efficacy, morbidity, and complications of the SMILE technique to radiofrequency reduction of the tongue base in adults with OSA. Although the effects of SMILE have shown promise, the SMILE technique is a relatively blind procedure and still difficult for most ear, nose, and throat surgeons. SMILE also resulted in some morbidity, such as damage to the lingual artery and hypoglossal nerve, and significant postoperative edema. Woodson[21] used coblation technique for tongue base resection under the assistance of direct laryngoscope for minimizing the risk of trauma and edema and to reduce morbidity. However, the operation view was very limited for the target lesion via the direct laryngoscope.

The authors further used the transoral Eco-TBR to treat hypopharyngeal collapse in OSA patients.[22] Their results demonstrated that transoral Eco-TBR resulted in short-term morbidity, and there were no serious long-term complications. They achieved reasonable surgical outcomes and ensured the safety of this procedure.

Because OSA is usually caused by multilevel obstructions, the true focus on efficacy should be on multilevel surgical intervention. The authors usually treated patients with modified UPPP combined with tongue base surgical modality, RFBOT for mild/moderate OSA and transoral Eco-TBR for moderate/severe OSA. The advantage of this minimally invasive REBOT procedure is that it can be repeated if the preliminary results are not satisfactory to physicians and patients.

TRANSORAL ROBOTIC SURGERY FOR OBSTRUCTIVE SLEEP APNEA

The da Vinci robotic system (Intuitive Surgical, Sunnyvale, CA, USA), with the angled scope and EndoWrist technology, allowed the sleep surgeon to deal with the angled corner of the tongue in the small oro-/hypopharyngeal cavity while maintaining agility and visibility of surgical area, thus allowing precise excision of the hypertrophic tongue tissue, lingual tonsils, and hypopharyngeal lesions.

In 2006, O'Malley and colleagues[23] first reported the use of transoral robotic surgery (TORS) for the upper aerodigestive tract neoplasms. In 2010, Vicini and colleagues[24] published the preliminary report on TORS for tongue base resection when treating OSA. They reported on their experience with TORS in the treatment of OSA, asserting its safety and efficacy in addressing obstruction at the BOT. There were clinical and cadaveric anatomic studies to help widespread use of this relatively new application in the surgical treatment of OSA. In 2012, Friedman and colleagues[25] presented the first report of TORS for the treatment of OSA in the United States. Their surgical cure rate for TORS was 66.7% in 40 consecutive patients with OSA. After that, Toh and colleagues[26] also presented the results of TORS for 20 patients with OSA in Asia in 2014. Their results showed that traditional cure (AHI <5/h) was achieved in 7 of 20 patients (35%), and traditional success was achieved in another 11 patients (55%).

After numerous reports on TORS for OSA, there were 3 systematic reviews and meta-analyses on TORS-assisted OSA surgery reports. The success rates were 48.2%,[27] 68.4%,[28] and 65.6%,[29] respectively.

BASE OF THE TONGUE SURGERY IN MULTILEVEL OBSTRUCTIVE SLEEP APNEA SURGERY

Because OSA is usually a result of multilevel obstructions of the upper airway and because many studies have demonstrated that multilevel treatment of all sites of obstruction lead to better surgical outcomes,[30] the combination of palatoplasty, septoplasty, and nonpacking endoscopic sinus surgery could be performed simultaneously with the above volumetric tongue base resection. For moderate/severe OSA patients who used CPAP preoperatively, they can continue to use CPAP immediately after surgery. In the authors' experience, this did not increase the complications of postoperative bleeding after minimally invasive or aggressive tongue base surgery.

OPERATIVE PREPARATION

Five days before the surgery, patients will begin to use 0.2% Chlorhexidine or 1% Povidone-iodine mouth rinses at least 2 times a day for oral hygiene. With the head mildly extended, exposure was obtained using a standard Jennings mouth gag retractor for RFBOT or Eco-TBR, and Crow Davis mouth gag and Davis Meyer tongue blade for TORS. The retention suture with 4-0 silk with taper needle could be settled down 1.5 cm anterior to the circumvallate papillae to increase the operative space of the obstructed tongue base region.

The REBOT and Eco-TBR was performed with the assistance of transoral 45° or 70° rigid sinus endoscope, depending on the angle of tongue base. TORS-assisted OSA surgery could be done with the da Vinci S/Si/Xi Surgical System. The authors used 30° Robotic Lens (12 mm, 8.5 mm), Maryland EndoWrist dissector (5 mm), and Monopolar Endowrist Cautery (5 mm).

When combined with nasal or palatal surgery, the authors suggest the volumetric tongue reduction as the last attempted procedure, because of concerns of damaging the tongue base wound and increasing the risk of postoperative bleeding from the base of the tongue.

ANESTHESIA

Regarding the type of intubation used on tongue base tissue volume reduction, most surgeons performed this procedure with transnasal endotracheal tube intubation. However, the authors favored the regular orotracheal intubation. The nasotracheal tube position usually induced inconvenience when performing the palatal and/or sinonasal surgeries simultaneously, if necessary. The other reason is the risk of compression damage of the nostril by the nasotracheal tube and increasing epistaxis when removing the tube. By using orotracheal intubation, the tube can be placed on one side of the mouth angle and the opposite side of the mouth can be fully exposed, which allows a better view when compared with the nasotracheal intubation. The apex of the inverted V-shape of the circumvallate papillae is the guide for the midline; it will not induce disorientation for the procedure. The only disadvantage of using an orotracheal tube in this procedure is the time used to change the tube to the opposite side of the mouth, although it usually only takes several seconds.

Patients are routinely extubated after fully recovering from the general anesthesia in the operation room. The authors do not have any experience with the complication of immediate acute airway obstruction, which needs to be reintubated, or acute tongue base wound bleeding after extubation in the operation room, up to now. Nasopharyngeal airway (nasal trump) should be available anytime if the patients develop signs of upper airway obstruction in the recovery room.

LINGUAL ARTERY ISSUE

Hou and colleagues[31] performed computed tomographic angiography (CTA) to determine the relationship between the lingual artery and lingual markers for preoperative evaluation of the lingual artery in 87 patients with OSA. Their results demonstrated that the course of the lingual artery with the tongue in a resting position was similar to that of the big dipper constellation in the sagittal view of CTA imaging. The first segment of the lingual artery declined approximately 19.3 ± 5.2 mm; the middle segment of the lingual artery was forward approximately 19.3 ± 6.8 mm, and the ascending segment of the lingual artery rose approximately 52.5 ± 10.9 mm. The entry point where the lingual artery entered into the tongue was adjacent to the tip of the greater horn of the hyoid bone. The relationship between the second segment of the lingual artery and the greater horn of the hyoid bone was relatively steady with the tongue in any position. The interval between the bilateral greater horn of the hyoid bone equaled that between the bilateral lingual arteries. In addition to transoral endoscope, recognizing the anatomic lingual markers in patients with OSA, such as the greater horn of the hyoid bone, foramen cecum, circumvallate papilla, lingual vein, and tongue midline, could facilitate the surgeon's ability to define the course of the lingual artery accurately and increase the surgical safety during these procedures.[31] Because vessel identification is always clear under the scopic guidance and the courses of the lingual artery have been well demonstrated,[32] the authors only used the handheld Doppler device in their first 10 patients with Eco-TBR to identify the courses of the neurovascular bundle.

POSTOPERATIVE CARE

Intravenous antibiotics (Cefazolin) were given perioperatively and postoperatively, and oral antibiotics (Cefadroxil) were used for 5 to 7 days after surgery. Intravenous steroids were prescribed for 5 days. Nonsteroidal anti-inflammatory drugs (Ibuprofen), proton pump inhibitor or H2-receptor antagonists, and 0.2% Chlorhexidine or 1% Povidone-iodine mouth rinses per the patient's request were prescribed for 1 week. Anti-inflammatory oral spray (benzydamine hydrochloride 1.5 mg/mL or 3 mg/mL) was used every 4 hours, if necessary. A liquid or soft diet was started 6 hours after the surgery.

COMPLICATIONS

Acute surgical complications of updated systematic review and meta-analysis on the effects of glossectomy as part of multilevel sleep surgery on OSA by Murphey and colleagues[6] only occurred in 16.4% (79/481) of reported patients. Complications arising from minimally invasive radiofrequency surgery to tongue base are rare and include ulceration or abscess formation, temporary tongue numbness, and lingual nerve paralysis. Most minor complications of volumetric tongue reduction encountered were related to postoperative throat discomfort, such as

sensation of a lump in the throat, dry throat, and frequent throat clearing. Patients usually did not think the above morbidity affected their social activities. Regarding postoperative bleeding that required surgical intervention, 1.7% to 5.5% was reported with TORS in the literature.[6] There were no reported cases of postoperative bleeding that required surgical intervention up to now in the authors' Eco-TBR, RF-BOT, and TORS series.

TASTE DISTURBANCE AFTER BASE OF THE TONGUE SURGERY

Up to July 2018, we have had 556 patients with OSA who underwent the treatment of the tongue base obstruction (unpublished data). There were no perioperative complications or cases of immediate postoperative airway obstruction or massive wound bleeding intheir case series. Most minor complications encountered were related to postoperative throat discomfort, such as pain, sensation of a lump in the throat, dry throat, and frequent throat clearing. No cases of hypoglossal nerve injury or permanent dysphagia were encountered in the authors' follow-up period. However, they did find that taste disturbance occurred in a subset of patients after OSA surgery. In 2016, they retrospectively investigated taste disturbance with a standard 3-drop-method gustatory function test following tongue base resection for the treatment of OSA.[33] At 3 months postoperative time, 8 (10%) of 80 patients still had changes in taste sensation; however, the taste disturbance severity decreased and did not impact the patients' regular social life. The percentage of taste change severity by time after tongue base surgery for OSA was between 13.8% and 17.5%. Thus, it is important to clearly inform the patient about the possibility of gustatory change after tongue base surgery for OSA preoperatively.

TREATMENT OPTIONS FOR FAILURE

The authors believe that facial box surgery, tongue base suspension procedures, or repeated tongue base tissue volume reduction might have a role in being the salvage technique for the failure of initial volumetric tongue reduction. Hypoglossal nerve stimulation may also be the alternative option for this treatment; however, the cost and possible morbidities of these alternatives still need to be considered. Furthermore, patients could definitely be advised to use the CPAP or oral appliance to treat the residual sleep apnea.

Based on the authors' experience, transoral volumetric tongue reduction has significant clinical benefits on the treatment of OSA patients with obvious tongue base obstruction. Their results have been encouraging overall up to now, and these procedures can be the surgical treatment of choice for OSA patients.

HIGHLIGHTS OF VOLUMETRIC TONGUE REDUCTION FOR OBSTRUCTIVE SLEEP APNEA

1. Select the adequate OSA patients for transoral tongue base volume reduction, such as a wide open mouth and good dentition.
2. Encourage oral hygiene before the surgery.
3. Precisely resect the hypertrophic tongue base and lingual tonsils tissues under clear scopic guidance.
4. Avoid damaging the dorsal branches of lingual arteries.
5. Adequate hemostasis with low-temperature device.
6. Raise the systolic blood pressure of the patient to greater than 100 mm Hg to check the wound status before finalizing the procedure.
7. A well-prepared surgical and anesthesia team to gently intubate and extubate the OSA patient for these procedures.

REFERENCES

1. Chabolle F, Wagner I, Blumen MB, et al. Tongue base reduction with hyoepiglottoplasty: a treatment for severe obstructive sleep apnea. Laryngoscope 1999;109:1273–80.
2. Kezirian EJ, Maselli J, Vittinghoff E, et al. Obstructive sleep apnea surgery practice patterns in the United States: 2000 to 2006. Otolaryngol Head Neck Surg 2010;143:441–7.
3. Kezirian EJ, Hussey HM, Brietzke SE, et al. Hypopharyngeal surgery in obstructive sleep apnea: practice patterns, perceptions, and attitudes. Otolaryngol Head Neck Surg 2012;147:964–71.
4. Brietzke SE, Ishman SL, Cohen S, et al. National database analysis of single-level versus multilevel sleep surgery. Otolaryngol Head Neck Surg 2017; 156:955–61.
5. Kezirian EJ, Goldberg AN. Hypopharyngeal surgery in obstructive sleep apnea: an evidence-based medicine review. Arch Otolaryngol Head Neck Surg 2006;132:206–13.
6. Murphey AW, Kandl JA, Nguyen SA, et al. The effect of glossectomy for obstructive sleep apnea: a systematic review and meta-analysis. Otolaryngol Head Neck Surg 2015;153:334–42.
7. Fujita S, Woodson BT, Clark JL, et al. Laser midline glossectomy as a treatment for obstructive sleep apnea. Laryngoscope 1991;101:805–9.
8. Prinsell JR. Maxillomandibular advancement surgery in a site-specific treatment approach for obstructive sleep apnea in 50 consecutive patients. Chest 1999;116:1519–29.
9. DeRowe A, Gunther E, Fibbi A, et al. Tongue-base suspension with a soft tissue-to-bone anchor for obstructive sleep apnea: preliminary clinical results of a new minimally invasive technique. Otolaryngol Head Neck Surg 2000;122:100–3.
10. Neruntarat C. Genioglossus advancement and hyoid myotomy: short-term and long-term results. J Laryngol Otol 2003;117:482–6.
11. Hörmann K, Baisch A. The hyoid suspension. Laryngoscope 2004;114:1677–9.
12. Friedman M, Tanyeri H, La Rosa M, et al. Clinical predictors of obstructive sleep apnea. Laryngoscope 1999;109:1901–7.
13. Friedman M, Ibrahim H, Bass L. Clinical staging for sleep-disordered breathing. Otolaryngol Head Neck Surg 2002;127:13–21.
14. Powell NB, Riley RW, Troell RJ, et al. Radiofrequency volumetric reduction of the soft palate in subjects with sleep-disordered breathing. Chest 1998;113: 1163–74.
15. Kotecha B. Updated minimally invasive surgery for sleep-related breathing disorders. Adv Otorhinolaryngol 2017;80:90–8.
16. Stimpson P, Kotecha B. Histopathological and ultrastructural effects of cutting radiofrequency energy on palatal soft tissues: a prospective study. Eur Arch Otorhinolaryngol 2011;268: 1829–36.
17. Powell NB, Riley RW, Guilleminault C. Radiofrequency tongue base reduction in sleep-disordered breathing: a pilot study. Otolaryngol Head Neck Surg 1999;120:656–64.
18. Babademez MA, Yorubulut M, Yurekli MF, et al. Comparison of minimally invasive techniques in tongue base surgery in patients with obstructive sleep apnea. Otolaryngol Head Neck Surg 2011; 145:858–64.
19. Friedman M, Soans R, Gurpinar B, et al. Evaluation of submucosal minimally invasive lingual excision technique for treatment of obstructive sleep apnea/hypopnea syndrome. Otolaryngol Head Neck Surg 2008;139:378–84.
20. Maturo SC, Mair EA. Submucosal minimally invasive lingual excision: an effective, novel surgery for pediatric tongue base reduction. Ann Otol Rhinol Laryngol 2006;115:624–30.
21. Woodson BT. Innovative technique for lingual tonsillectomy and midline posterior glossectomy for obstructive sleep apnea. Oper Tech Otolaryngol Head Neck Surg 2007;18:20–8.
22. Lin HC, Friedman M, Chang HW, et al. ZPPP combined with endoscopic coblator open tongue base resection for severe obstructive sleep apnea/

hypopnea syndrome. Otolaryngol Head Neck Surg 2014;150:1078–85.

23. O'Malley BW Jr, Weinstein GS, Snyder W, et al. Transoral robotic surgery (TORS) for base of tongue neoplasms. Laryngoscope 2006;116:1465–72.

24. Vicini C, Dallan I, Canzi P, et al. Transoral robotic tongue base resection in obstructive sleep apnoea-hypopnoea syndrome: a preliminary report. ORL J Otorhinolaryngol Relat Spec 2010;72:22–7.

25. Friedman M, Hamilton C, Samuelson CG, et al. Transoral robotic glossectomy for the treatment of obstructive sleep apnea-hypopnea syndrome. Otolaryngol Head Neck Surg 2012;146:854–62.

26. Toh ST, Han HJ, Tay HN, et al. Transoral robotic surgery for obstructive sleep apnea in Asian patients: a Singapore sleep centre experience. JAMA Otolaryngol Head Neck Surg 2014;140:624–9.

27. Justin GA, Chang ET, Camacho M, et al. Transoral robotic surgery for obstructive sleep apnea: a systematic review and meta-analysis. Otolaryngol Head Neck Surg 2016;154:835–46.

28. Miller SC, Nguyen SA, Ong AA, et al. Transoral robotic base of tongue reduction for obstructive sleep apnea: a systematic review and meta-analysis. Laryngoscope 2017;127:258–65.

29. Meccariello G, Cammaroto G, Montevecchi F, et al. Transoral robotic surgery for the management of obstructive sleep apnea: a systematic review and meta-analysis. Eur Arch Otorhinolaryngol 2017;274:647–53.

30. Lin HC, Friedman M, Chang HW, et al. The efficacy of multilevel surgery of the upper airway in adults with obstructive sleep apnea/hypopnea syndrome. Laryngoscope 2008;118:902–28.

31. Hou TN, Zhou LN, Hu HJ. Computed tomographic angiography study of the relationship between the lingual artery and lingual markers in patients with obstructive sleep apnoea. Clin Radiol 2011;66:526–9.

32. Woodson BT, Laohasiriwong S. Lingual tonsillectomy and midline posterior glossectomy for obstructive sleep apnea. Oper Tech Otolaryngol Head Neck Surg 2012;23:155–61.

33. Lin HC, Hwang MS, Liao CC, et al. Taste disturbance following tongue base resection for OSA. Laryngoscope 2016;126:1009–13.

Transoral Robotic Surgery for Obstructive Sleep Apnea: Past, Present, and Future

Claudio Vicini, MD[a,b], Filippo Montevecchi, MD[b],*

KEYWORDS

- OSA • Robotic • Sleep apnea • Orohypopharyngeal • Tracheostomy • Vallecula

KEY POINTS

- Nocturnal upper airway collapse often involves the obstruction at the tongue base.
- Several surgical procedures have been developed in recent years to address this area in continuous positive airway pressure-nonadherent patients and include hyolingual advancement, tongue suture suspension, and various lingual resection techniques.
- Traditional tongue base resection is generally done either via a transcervical technique or transorally with an endoscope for visualization.
- Each of these approaches has significant potential limitations.
- The unsurpassed visualization, dexterity, and control provided by the Da Vinci Surgical System offer many benefits for the surgeon compared with the other technologies.

INTRODUCTION

Trans oral robotic surgery (TORS) refers to a variety of procedures using the da Vinci Surgical System produced by Intuitive Surgical Inc, Sunnyvale, CA. Collectively, TORS procedures involve the precise endoscopic excision of oral, orohypopharyngeal, and laryngeal tissue with a variety of articulated, wristed instruments placed alongside a 3-dimensional (3D), high-definition endoscopic camera, all controlled by the surgeon from a remote operating room console. TORS was pioneered by Weinstein and O'Malley at Penn University as a minimally invasive technique for treatment of oropharyngeal cancers and was approved by Food and Drug Administration for adult head and neck surgery in December, 2009. It has since become adopted worldwide and is considered by many practitioners to be the most effective and reproducible minimally invasive surgical technique available. The unsurpassed visualization, dexterity, and control provided by the da Vinci offer the following benefits for the surgeon: superior exposure and 3D HD visualization of the target anatomy inside the pharynx, more precise dissection and improved preservation of intralingual vessels and nerves, shorter learning curve, faster operative time, and a more reproducible approach as compared with traditional open as well as endoscopic techniques.[1–5] It also offers significant patient benefits: excellent cosmetic outcomes, no neck scars (except for tracheostomy, if necessary),[6,7] reduced likelihood of iatrogenic injury to vessels and nerves, better and faster functional recovery compared with the transcervical approach, reduced operating room time, and shortened length of hospital stay. Tongue base reduction (TBR) refers to the primary focus of this targeted surgery for obstructive sleep apnea (OSA): "a robotic-assisted resection of a part of the base of the tongue from roughly the foramen cecum to the vallecula." Note that in the context of sleep-

[a] Otolaryngology–Head and Neck Surgery, University of Ferrara, Via Aldo Moro 8, Ferrara 44124, Italy; [b] Head and Neck Department, ENT & Oral Surgery Unit, G.B. Morgagni - L. Pierantoni Hospital, ASL of Romagna, Via Carlo Forlanini 34, Forlì 47100, Italy
* Corresponding author.
E-mail addresses: filippomontevecchi72@gmail.com; filo651@hotmail.com

Sleep Med Clin 14 (2019) 67–72
https://doi.org/10.1016/j.jsmc.2018.10.008
1556-407X/19/© 2018 Elsevier Inc. All rights reserved.

disordered breathing, the term "reduction" is preferred to "resection," a term usually associated with cancer applications. TBR can include removal of lingual tonsillar tissue, tongue base musculature, or both. The amount of resection can vary from several milliliter to greater than 50 mL as needed, based on the patient's anatomy and degree of prolapse during sleep. Irrespective to histology or volume of the resected tissue, the goal is to clear the airway. Supraglottoplasty (SGP) refers to the adjunctive treatment of collapsible epiglottic, arytenoids, and/or aryepiglottic tissue. The suffix "plasty" intentionally includes broad range of surgical manipulations of such floppy supraglottic tissue and is tailored to the presenting pathology.

EXPOSURE

The patient is positioned supine in the sniffing position (neck flexed and head extended) in order to achieve the best exposure. External compression maneuvers can be used in order to enhance the exposure of different areas during the dissection (hyoid compression or other manoeuvers). Tongue base exposure is achieved in the standard TORS approach with a combination of tongue tip traction (with a 0 silk stitch horizontal mattress suture) and tongue body displacement by Storz, Davis-Meyer mouth gag under direct visualization with a head light. A complete set of tongue blades of different sizes with integrated suction tubes (for smoke and blood) is of paramount importance. A small, wide blade has proved to be the most suitable tool in most cases (Storz blade number 1 and 2) (Storz Cat. 743910 and 743920). At the end of the exposure the tip of the blade is just anterior to the circumvallate papillae (**Fig. 1**). In patients with significant macroglossia the smaller and narrower blade may cause significant lateral in-rolling of the tongue body margins. In this situation the

working space will be reduced and the introduction of the robotic arms may be difficult. The use of a longer and wider blade (Storz blade number 3) (Storz Cat. 743930) is possible in order to prevent lateral tongue body prolapse into the surgical field. In cases of macroglossia the tongue is partially released in order to allow adequate exposure of the tongue base. A combination of tongue base traction and properly selected mouth-gag blade length is the key for excellent exposure. Repositioning of the tongue blade during the resection is rarely necessary. Usually the short or the medium blade (Storz blade number 1 and 2) are very effective for completing tongue base as well as epiglottis procedures. If a second blade is to be inserted after the initial resection, the new position must be carefully verified in order to avoid the loss of proper orientation. The 12-mm 30° 3D scope (upward facing) is our preferred choice. If available an 8-mm scope may be very helpful in particular cases (minimal interincisive distance, extreme macroglossia, etc.). Only 2 robotic 5-mm Endo Wrist are routinely used for each patient: a Maryland Dissector for grasping and dissecting tissues and a monopolar cautery with a spatula tip for dissection and coagulation. Surgical clip placement is usually not required, but in special cases clipping of large vessels may prove to be very helpful. Additional hemostasis can be provided by using an insulated coagulation-suction tube, Storz Cat. 12067R. An insulated bipolar forceps, Storz Cat. 842219, is of paramount importance for safe coagulation in the peripheral aspects of the surgical field. The forceps must be insulated from the tip to the handle in order to avoid burns of the oral commissure. A Neurosurgical Malis Bipolar (Codman) or a bipolar Dessi (Microfrance) coagulating device originally studied for sinus surgery may be helpful as well. The bedside assistant provides 2 additional suction devices (Lawton suction Cat. 160274), which can be used for retraction and the evacuation of smoke and blood.

SURGICAL STEPS

TORS approach for OSA may include 2 different surgical steps frequently combined in the same procedures according to the patient's features: tongue base reduction and supraglottoplasty.[8–10]

Tongue Base Reduction

The goal of TBR is to enlarge the oropharyngeal space by removing tissue from the anterior wall. The end point of TBR may be achieved when the surgical view changes from a Cormack & Lehane Grade IV or III to a Grade II or I.[11,12] In most cases

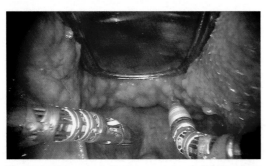

Fig. 1. At the end of the exposure the tip of the blade is anterior to the circumvallate papillae. In the surgical field there are 2 robotic instruments, a Maryland forcep and a monopolar cautery.

lymphoid tissue as well as tongue base muscle must be removed in order to clear the retrolingual space or posterior airway space. In case of massive lymphoid hyperplasia less muscular tissue needs to be removed. Conversely, if the lingual tonsils are not enlarged then a more aggressive muscular resection is required in order to obtain the Cormack & Lehane Grade II/I. The mean volume of tissue removed is typically 10 mL, but in some cases the overall volume may be up to 50 mL. The surgical steps are standardized in a precise and logical sequence and will be described in detail.

Right-side lingual tonsillectomy

Instrument setting:
    Maryland left
    Monopolar right
    Setting: coagulation/blended (no cutting)
    Energy level (15–30) according to the device

The procedure starts with a midline split of the 2 lingual tonsils from foramen caecum in order to identify the tip of epiglottis and vallecula (**Fig. 2**). The dissection is carried out using monopolar cautery until the junction between lymphatic tissue and muscle is identified. In patients with extreme lingual tonsil hypertrophy it may be difficult to identify the foramen caecum and circumvallate papilla. In these cases debulking of the midline lymphoid tissue may help the surgeon to identify the essential surgical landmarks. At the beginning of the dissection it is strongly recommended that the surgeon position the tip of the scope far from the tongue base in order to provide a wide surgical view under low magnification; this will enhance the surgeon's 3D awareness of the anatomy. At the end of this first step, the lingual tonsils are completely divided in the midline creating a deep groove joining the foramen caecum superiorly to the glossoepiglottic ligament inferiorly. Dissection is carried out using the tip of the spatula, "painting"

layer by layer through the tissue in order to maintain direct visualization of the tip of the instrument. In order to grasp the tissue a deep cut must be created to allow the Maryland forceps to gain adequate purchase of the tissue, otherwise repeated attempts of grasping will produce tedious, excessive bleeding (**Fig. 3**). In cases of mild to moderate lingual tonsil hyperplasia, after midline dissection, the superior (sulcus terminalis), lateral (glossotonsillar sulcus), and inferior (glossoepiglottic sulcus) borders of the right lingual tonsil are identified and marked by cautery. In cases of extreme lingual tonsil hyperplasia, after midline splitting, it is recommended to perform a midline lingual tonsil debulking in order to allow better manipulation and better identification of the limit of the dissection. If lingual tonsil hyperplasia is mild to moderate, the right lingual tonsillectomy is performed "en block" superiorly to inferiorly maintaining the dissection plane close to the lympho-muscular junction. During this step the scope is positioned closer to the surgical field for better identification of neurovascular structures. Bleeding during this phase of the dissection is usually minimal. Additional remarks include the following:

- A precise multidimensional resection is easily performed with the 3D view of the Da Vinci optics.
- Bedside assistant maintains countertraction in order to assist the surgeon during dissection; increased tension allows more precise and quicker dissection (**Fig. 4**).
- The inferior limit of the resection is characterized by a bluish color representing the vallecular mucosa and by an increased bleeding.

Left-side lingual tonsillectomy

Instrument setting:
    Maryland right
    Monopolar left

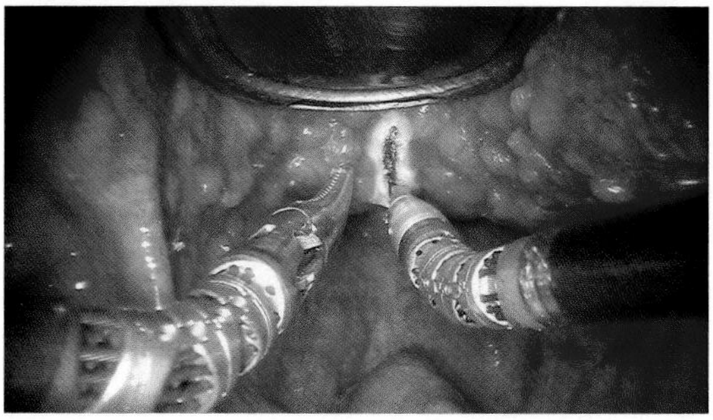

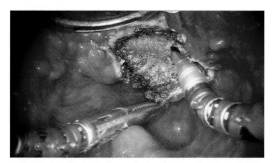

Fig. 2. The procedure starts with a midline split of the 2 lingual tonsils from foramen caecum in order to identify the tip of epiglottis and vallecula.

Fig. 3. In order to grasp the tissue a deep cut must be created to allow the Maryland forceps to gain adequate purchase of the tissue.

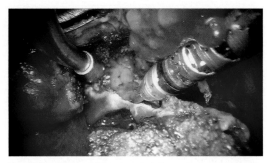

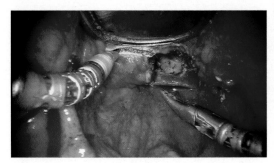

Fig. 4. Bedside assistant maintains countertraction in order to assist the surgeon during dissection; increased tension allows more precise and quicker dissection.

Fig. 6. Left lingual tonsillectomy is completed in the same way as that of the right after side inversion of the robotic arms and tools. Initial mucosa dissection.

Setting: coagulation/blended (no cutting)
Energy level (15–30) according to the device

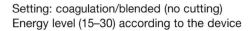

After completing right lingual tonsillectomy (**Fig. 5**), left lingual tonsillectomy is completed in the same way after side inversion of the robotic arms and tools (**Figs. 6–8**).

Residual obstruction evaluation

The surgical field is now inspected in order to evaluate the residual degree of obstruction. If Cormack & Lehane Grade is greater than 2, additional resection in the muscle layer is required. Additional information is provided by the volume of tissue resected and measured using a graduated syringe filled with saline. If the overall volume of resected tissue is less than 7 mL an additional resection may be recommended. Repositioning of the tongue blade or replacement of the tongue blade with a larger and or smaller blade may assist the surgeon by exposing tissue that may have been compressed by the retractor.

Additional resections

In order to open the posterior airway space it may be necessary to remove muscle in addition to lymphoid tissue. When entering the muscular layer it is important to avoid injury to the neurovascular structures, including the dorsal branches of the lingual arteries and hypoglossal nerve. Several investigators have published interesting cadaveric dissections[10,13–15] describing practical anatomic landmarks in this area. Woodson stresses the importance of intraoperative mapping of the tongue vasculature using ultrasound if available. Most investigators would agree that anatomic landmarks are unreliable due to great individual anatomic variability and the extreme mobility of the active tongue. In addition, the tongue shape is modified in the surgical setting due to retraction and positioning.[16] In the authors' experience 2 additional points must be stressed:

- The relationship of the lingual artery and hyoid bone is a reliable landmark.[10]
- The 3D HD Da Vinci camera allows for the identification of the crucial structures before damaging them, working carefully step by step, with a mix of blunt and sharp dissection.

The overall time required for TBR is about 30 minutes.

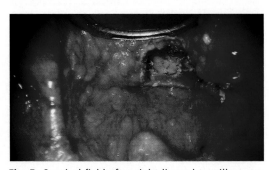

Fig. 5. Surgical field after right lingual tonsillectomy.

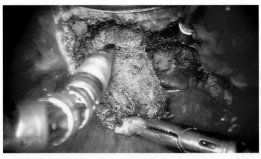

Fig. 7. Left lingual tonsillectomy is completed in the same way as that of the right after side inversion of the robotic arms and tools. Dissection of deeper layers.

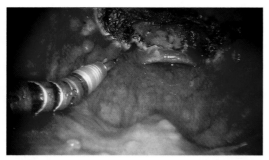

Fig. 8. Surgical field at the end of the lingual tonsillectomy. At this step a view of the epiglottis is possible.

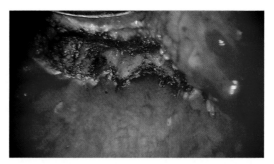

Fig. 10. Surgical field at the end of the epiglottoplasty.

Supraglottoplasty

Supraglottoplasty may be carried out concurrent with TBR in patient with primary and in some cases secondary epiglottic collapse. The role of SGP is to prevent the inward collapse of the floppy epiglottis and/or redundant supraglottic tissue. The additional time required for SPG is usually less than 15 minutes. The most common procedure in supraglottic area includes the following steps:

- *Vertical midline splitting of supra-hyoid epiglottis*: this step is carried out along the midline, following the medial glossoepiglottic fold, from the tip of the epiglottis inferiorly, preserving at least 5 mm of epiglottis above the deep vallecular plane (a sufficient remnant of epiglottic cartilage is left to avoid aspiration).
- *A horizontal section is performed bilaterally* in a plane joining the vertical section in the midline and running laterally immediately over the pharyngoepiglottic fold, in order to leave a lateral fold preventing aspiration, and in order to avoid possible bleeding from the superior laryngeal vessels (**Figs. 9** and **10**). Scarring of the vallecular and perivallecular area leads to progressive adhesion and stabilization of the residual epiglottis to the tongue base.

- A modification of the previously described procedure as described by Magnuson (unpublished data) is the "V-shape" epiglottoplasty. A V-shape wedge is removed from the central epiglottis. This technique it is probably safer for the airway and for the superior laryngeal vascular bundle.

The surgical steps shown in **Figs. 9** and **10** have been performed in patients who have undergone planned preoperative tracheostomy. Tracheostomy is not performed routinely for patients undergoing TORS but is performed in certain circumstances: (1) patients who were found to have a difficult intubation and (2) situations where emergent reintubation is anticipated to be difficult. It is important to understand that tracheostomy is not performed solely due to an enlarged tongue base. In most cases, surgeon preference dictates either transnasal or transoral intubation for benign base of tongue TORS procedures. Consultation with the anesthesia provider about the possibility of tracheostomy should be discussed both before and after intubation. Although unplanned tracheostomy is rare, patients should be aware and consented for this possibility.[17]

SUMMARY

Traditional surgery to address base of tongue obstruction during sleep has significant limitations. Although many patients benefit from the use of continuous positive airway pressure therapy, noncompliant patients require a surgical procedure to eliminate the obstruction. TORS for OSA allows the surgeon to address the base of tongue obstruction with several advantages. The minimally invasive procedure is well tolerated by the patient. In the future, a new generation of robotic tools may be dedicated for OSA surgery and perhaps revolutionary robotic systems will be available. New instrumentation including retractors and blades will improve exposure, and alternative cutting devices may improve postoperative

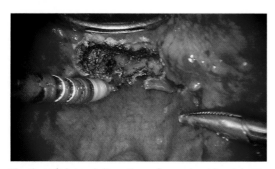

Fig. 9. Left lateral dissection of suprahyoid epiglottis.

morbidity. A navigation system may allow surgeons to plan and carry out surgery with more precision. Tissue specific dyes will be available for easier intraoperative identification of nerves and vessels.

REFERENCES

1. Fujita S, Woodson BT, Clark JL, et al. Laser midline glossectomy as a treatment for obstructive sleep apnea. Laryngoscope 1991;101(8):805–9.

2. Mickelson S, Rosenthal L. Midline glossectomy and epiglottidectomy for obstructive sleep apnea syndrome. Laryngoscope 1997;107(5):614–9.

3. Chabolle F, Wagner I, Blumen MB, et al. Tongue base reduction with hyoepigottoplasty: a treatment for severe obstructive sleep apnea. Laryngoscope 1999;109(8):1273–80.

4. Blumen MB, Coquille F, Rocchicioli C, et al. Radiofrequency tongue reduction through a cervical approach: a pilot study. Laryngoscope 2006; 116(10):1887–93.

5. Friedman M, Soans R, Gurpinar B, et al. Evaluation of submucosal minimally invasive lingual excision technique for treatment of obstructive sleep apnea/hypopnea syndrome. Otolaryngol Head Neck Surg 2008;139(3):378–84.

6. Campanini A, De Vito A, Frassineti S, et al. Temporary tracheotomy in the surgical treatment of obstructive sleep apnea syndrome: personal experience. Acta Otorhinolaryngol Ital 2003;23(6):474–8.

7. Sun H, Lou W, Wang L, et al. Clinical significance of preoperative tracheotomy in preventing perioperative OSAHS severe complications. Lin Chuang Er Bi Yan Hou Ke Za Zhi 2005;19(9):394–5.

8. Vicini C, Dallan I, Canzi P, et al. Transoral robotic tongue base resection in obstructive sleep apnoea-hypopnoea syndrome: a preliminary report. ORL J Otorhinolaryngol Relat Spec 2010;72(1):22–7.

9. Vicini C, Montevecchi F, Tenti G, et al. Transoral robotic surgery: tongue base reduction and supraglottoplasty for obstructive sleep apnea. Original research article. Oper Tech Otolayngol Head Neck Surg 2012;23(1):45–7.

10. Vicini C, Dallan I, Canzi P, et al. Transoral robotic surgery of the tongue base in obstructive sleep Apnea-Hypopnea syndrome: anatomic considerations and clinical experience. Head Neck 2012;34:15–22.

11. Cormack RS, Lehane J. Difficult tracheal intubation in obstetrics. Anaesthesia 1984;39(11):1105–11.

12. Yentis SM, Lee DJ. Evaluation of an improved scoring system for the grading of direct laryngoscopy. Anaesthesia 1998;53(11):1041–4.

13. Sequert C, Lestang P, Baglin AC, et al. Hypoglossal nerve in its intralingual trajectory: anatomy and clinical implications. Ann Otolaryngol Chir Cervicofac 1999;116(4):207–17.

14. Lauretano AM, Li KK, Caradonna DS, et al. Anatomic location of the tongue base neurovascular bundle. Laryngoscope 1997;107(8):1057–9.

15. O'Malley BW Jr, Weinstein GS, Snyder W, et al. Transoral robotic surgery (TORS) for base of tongue neoplasms. Laryngoscope 2006;116(8):1465–72.

16. Wu D, Qin J, Guo X, et al. Analysis of the difference in the course of the lingual arteries caused by tongue position change. Laryngoscope 2015; 125(3):762–6.

17. Vicini C, Hoff P, Montevecchi F, editors. TransOral robotic surgery for obstructive sleep apnea. Switzerland: Springer; 2016. ISBN: 978-3-319-34038-8 (Print) 978-3-319-34040-1 (Online).

Genioglossus Advancement and Hyoid Surgery

Yau Hong Goh, MD, PhD[a], Victor Abdullah, MD, PhD[b],
Sung Wan Kim, MD, PhD[c],*

KEYWORDS

- Obstructive sleep apnea • Genioglossus advancement • Hyoid surgery

KEY POINTS

- The structure and dimensions of the mandible, tongue, and hyoid complex are important variables in the pathophysiology of obstructive sleep apnea (OSA) at the hypopharyngeal level.
- Genioglossus advancement is based on mandibular osteotomy, which brings the genioglossus muscle forward and prevents posterior collapse during sleep.
- The hyoid surgery on the hypopharynx and tongue obstruction have played an important role in the development of surgery for OSA.

ANATOMIC CONSIDERATIONS

Tongue Musculature

The muscles of the tongue are grouped into intrinsic and extrinsic muscles (**Fig. 1**). Whereas the extrinsic muscles have bony attachments, intrinsic muscles are wholly within the tongue and are not attached to bony structures. Separated by a midline fibrous septum, each half of the tongue comprises 4 intrinsic muscles: the superior and inferior longitudinal muscles, as well as the transverse and vertical tongue muscles. These muscles enable the 3-dimensional manipulation of tongue shape during mastication and speech. The extrinsic muscle group comprises the hyoglossus, styloglossus, palatoglossus, and genioglossus muscles (GGM). Of these, the GGM is the largest and constitutes the primary mass of the tongue. As the names imply, these extrinsic muscles have attachments to the hyoid bone, styloid process, palatine aponeurosis, and genial tubercle (GT) of the mandible, respectively.

The GGM originates from the GT in the inner table of the mandible and its extensions are woven into the mucous membrane of the tongue. The inferior-most muscle fibers extend directly to the hyoid bone. The entire tongue mass lies on and is supported by the mylohyoid.

The mylohyoid is a thin sheet of muscle that forms the diaphragm of the floor of mouth. The mylohyoid muscle fibers span downward and medially from the mylohyoid line of the mandible into a midline raphe; the posterior quarter of these fibers is inserted into the body of the hyoid bone. The mylohyoid is arranged in a manner similar to that of the levator ani in the pelvic floor. However, unlike the levator ani, which has a midline raphe that is attached to a fixed bony anchor (the tip of

---

Disclosure Statement: The authors report no commercial or financial associations that might pose or create conflict with information presented in the article.

[a] Department of Otorhinolaryngology–Head and Neck Surgery, Mount Elizabeth Medical Centre, 3 Mount Elizabeth, Suite 03-01/02, Singapore 228510, Singapore; [b] Department of Otorhinolaryngology, Head and Neck Surgery (ENT), Chinese University of Hong Kong, United Christian Hospital, Room 26, B4, Block S, No. 130, Hip Wo Street, Kwun Tong, Kowloon, Hong Kong, China; [c] Department of Otorhinolaryngology–Head and Neck Surgery, Kyung Hee University Hospital, 23 Kyungheedae-ro, Dongdaemun-gu, Seoul 02447, Korea
* Corresponding author.
E-mail address: drkimsw@hanmail.net

Sleep Med Clin 14 (2019) 73–81
https://doi.org/10.1016/j.jsmc.2018.10.009
1556-407X/19/© 2018 Elsevier Inc. All rights reserved.

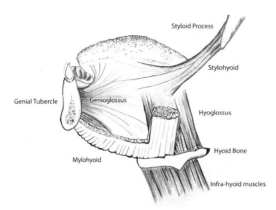

Fig. 1. A diagrammatic depiction of the mandible, key tongue musculature, and the hyoid bone complex.

the coccyx), the mylohyoid raphe is attached posteriorly to the mobile hyoid bone. The hypermobility of the hyoid bone (movement in an anterior-posterior manner, as well as a vertical manner) makes the floor of the mouth much more movable than the pelvic floor. This facilitates a greater range of mobility for the already flexible tongue.

As a predominantly muscular organ, the overall muscle tone of the tongue therefore affects the placement of the hyoid bone and the volume of the hypopharyngeal passage. Factors that lower the tonal quality of tongue muscles, such as alcohol/sedative consumption, anesthesia, and hypotonic state during rapid eye movement sleep, adversely affect the upper airway space.

Interspersed within the tongue mass is a variable quantity of adipose tissue. In a comparison of patients with and without apneas (matched for body mass index, gender, and age), the volume and the fat content within the tongue were increased in patients with apneas, compared with controls. This increased tongue-fat content in obese persons may explain the association between weight gain and obstructive sleep apnea (OSA).[1] Weight loss has also been shown to reduce tongue volume and fat content.

The Hyoid Bone

The hyoid bone is suspended between the mandible and styloid process by 2 muscle-straps: the geniohyoid and stylohyoid muscles. The alternating and reciprocal contractions of these 2 muscles determine the anteroposterior location of the hyoid bone. In conjunction with the mylohyoid and geniohyoid, the stylohyoid elevates the hyoid bone, whereas infrahyoid muscles depress the hyoid bone in a reciprocating manner.

Concept of Genioglossus Advancement and Hyoid Surgery

The structure and dimensions of the mandible, tongue, and hyoid complex are important variables in the pathophysiology of OSA at the hypopharyngeal level.[2,3] Airway collapse at the hypopharynx-tongue base level and the loss of muscle tone of pharyngeal dilators are major contributory factors in the onset of OSA. The hyoid bone and its muscle attachments affect hypopharyngeal airway resistance and patency.

The rationale for surgical interventions at the tongue base is to reduce the posterior displacement of structures in the region during sleep.[4,5] Genioglossus advancement (GA) and hyoid surgery primarily target the muscle tension of the tongue and limit its posterior collapse during sleep, especially in the supine position. However, unlike the more the radical maxillomandibular advancement technique, the degree of expansion in hypopharyngeal space achieved by GA and hyoid surgery is relatively limited. The scope of the procedures is restricted by the extent of forward advancement of the GT (the thickness of the body of mandible) and the degree of anterior movement of the hyoid bone. Commonly performed in combination with uvulopalatopharyngoplasty, GGM and hyoid surgeries have undergone multiple revisions and improvements over nearly 3 decades. The clinical effects and long-term benefits continue to be investigated.

GENIOGLOSSUS ADVANCEMENT

GA is a popular procedure for the treatment of tongue base level in OSA. This procedure is based on mandibular osteotomy, which brings the GGM forward and prevents posterior collapse during sleep.[6] However, the efficacy of GA is variable and inconstant as a result of both indication bias and the surgical technique.

The GA technique was firstly introduced by Powell and colleagues[7] in 1983 during sliding osteotomy with bilateral sagittal split osteotomy (BSSO). It was modified into the inferior sagittal osteotomy in 1986.[8] However, there was a high risk of mandible fracture after surgery; hence, the approach for GA was converted to a rectangular osteotomy of the mandible in 1993.[9] Diverse modifications have since enhanced surgical effectiveness and minimized the side effects. Mandibular trapezoid osteotomy to advance the GGM was reported in 1998.[10] The elliptical window GA was introduced by Dattilo and Aynechi,[11] and the trephine osteotomy approach was developed from a simpler surgical technique.[12] Hendler and colleagues[13] reported mortised genioplasty to advance the GGM more effectively, and Garcia Vega and colleagues[14] recently reported modified GA techniques that compensated for the disadvantages of rectangular osteotomy. **Table 1** summarizes the characteristics of these procedures (**Fig. 2**).

The GA technique has recently undergone several modifications; each has attempted to minimize surgical morbidity while improving the incorporation and advancement of the GGM.[15,16] Adequate advancement of the GT is believed to be most important for maximization of the surgical effect.[6,8,15–17] Therefore, osteotomy positioning is important for this purpose; however, there have been insufficient studies to provide a precise understanding of optimal positioning. Among these various transformations, the most fundamental requirements for determining the appropriate osteotomy location are precise knowledge of the GT location and the site of GGM origin. The GT is typically identified intraoperatively by finger palpation of the floor of the mouth and with the aid of

preoperative imaging studies.[17] Preoperative radiographs enable estimation of the location of the GT. There have been multiple efforts to determine the location of the GT by using cephalometry,[17,18] but these have been difficult due to limited images. According to recent research with 3-dimensional computed tomography (3D CT), the location of the GT varies in each case.[19] It has also been proven that GA surgery may not be appropriate for some patients due to anatomical-structural limits.[19] Previous studies have shown that there is no difference in GT width, depending on the angle or curvature of the mandible; however, positions along the height of the upper margin may differ between outer and inner tables.[17,18] Notably, 3D CT can be used to measure the position or size of the GT solely on the inner table of the mandible.[19] Preoperative radiographs help to estimate the location of the GT. Therefore, the results of previous imaging studies with 3D CT have some limitations when applied to actual operations, because osteotomy is performed by assuming the position of the GT, based on the outer table of the mandible

Table 1
Summary of characteristics of various genioglossus advancement techniques

1st Author, Year	Name of Surgical Technique	Advantages	Disadvantages
Powell et al,[7] 1983	BSSO		High risk of mandible fracture after surgery
Riley et al,[8] 1986	Inferior mandibular sagittal osteotomy		High risk of mandible fracture after surgery
Riley et al,[9] 1993	Rectangular osteotomy	Low risk of mandible fracture, short operation time	Difficult to confirm the location of GT, control of bleeding, and control of the degree of advancement of the GT
Dattilo,[10] 1998	Mandibular trapezoid osteotomy	Can advance the entire GGM	Can cause facial deformity, high risk of mandible fracture
Dattilo & Aynechi,[11] 2007	Elliptical window GA	Very low risk of mandible fracture	Complicated procedure, difficult to control of the degree of advancement of the GT
Miller et al,[12] 2004	Trephine osteotomy approach	Simple procedure	Poor accuracy
Hendler et al,[13] 2001	Mortised genioplasty	More effective advancement of GGM	Relatively high risk of mandible fracture
Garcia Vega et al,[14] 2014	Modified GA technique	Minimized muscle damage	Complicated procedure, difficult to apply for small mandible

Abbreviations: BSSO, bilateral sagittal split osteotomy; GA, genioglossus advancement; GGM, genioglossus muscle; GT, genial tubercle.

Data from Jung SY, Eun YG, Min JY, et al. Anatomical analysis to establish the optimal positioning of an osteotomy for genioglossal advancement-a trial in cadavers. Br J Oral Maxillofac Surg 2018;56(8):671–7.

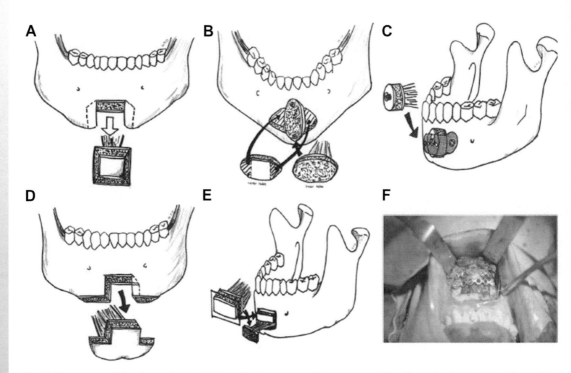

Fig. 2. Various modifications of GA. (*A*) Mandibular trapezoid osteotomy, (*B*) elliptical window GA, (*C*) trephine osteotomy approach, (*D*) mortised genioplasty, (*E*) modified geniotubercle advancement, (*F*) anterior mandibular segmental advancement.

during GA. Hence, there might be visible differences in the operative field that could help to determine the optimal positioning of the osteotomy on the outer table.[17,18,20]

Among the various procedures performed in GA, the most difficult positioning technique is superior horizontal osteotomy, which may cause undesirable complications, such as dental root damage of the lower incisor.[21] When it is not adequately elevated, the GT may be cut separately or excluded, which may have a critical effect on the surgical outcome.[12,19] Therefore, the proper positioning of these superior horizontal osteotomies during GA is an essential and important process to reduce the complications of surgery and achieve the desired effect. According to a recent cadaveric trial, an osteotomy that includes the GT may be possible in most patients when the osteotomy is positioned 2 mm higher, at the superior border of the GT to the inferior border of the mandible (SGT-IBM), than the location estimated from the inner table (**Fig. 3**).[22] To apply these

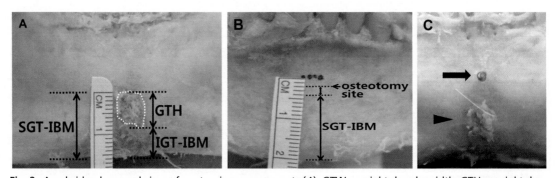

Fig. 3. An abridged general view of anatomic measurements (*A*). GTW, genial tubercle width; GTH, genial tubercle height; IGT-IBM, distance from the inferior border of the genial tubercle to the inferior border of the mandible. (*B*) Drilling site, a hole was drilled in the outer table of the mandible, 2 mm higher than the SGT-IBM of the inner table. (*C*) Drilling did not penetrate (*arrow*) the GT (*arrowhead*). (*Data from* Jung SY, Eun YG, Min JY, et al. Anatomical analysis to establish the optimal positioning of an osteotomy for genioglossal advancement-a trial in cadavers. Br J Oral Maxillofac Surg 2018;56(8):671–7.)

results to actual surgery, it is necessary to measure the SGT-IBM in the inner table. This can be accomplished with various imaging studies, including cephalometry and 3D CT.[17–19] In particular, agreement between the actual sizes of various landmarks of mandible and measurements obtained from 3D CT is reported to be quite high.[23] Further, the surgeon can measure SGT-IBM values from the 3D CT, as previously described.[19] Therefore, safe and accurate GA (including the whole GT) can be achieved when osteotomy is performed slightly above than the position of SGT-IBM obtained from the measurement at the inner table of the 3D CT.[22]

Recently, virtual simulation surgery has been used to implement an accurate GA technique.[24] In this process, after making a 3D image of the mandible, it is possible to perform a bone cut with any plane. Then, the surgeon can check whether GT is included, and can move the cut fragment from the mandible, exactly as the surgeon wishes; the amount of advancement can be checked, and a template of the osteotomy guide can be made with the 3D printing technique for real surgery (**Fig. 4**). During real surgery, the 3D template prepared in the simulation process can be placed in the mandible of the patient and guided osteotomy can be performed along the margin of the template. In addition, advancement of bone fragments isolated from the mandible can be appropriately controlled through osteotomy by using prefabricated fixation plates and screws designed during simulated surgery (**Fig. 5**). These virtual simulation surgeries have helped to overcome the disadvantages of conventional GA procedures. After using virtual simulation techniques and possible precise osteotomy approaches, we may obtain better anatomic and physiologic candidates for GA.

HYOID SURGERY IN OBSTRUCTIVE SLEEP APNEA

The hyoid bone has been of interest in sleep apnea and apnea-related surgical procedures because of its integral relationship with the tongue base and hypopharynx. It is a horseshoe-shaped floating bone without articulation, solely with muscle attachments. The hyoid bone provides an anchor for the tongue base. Muscles attached to the hyoid bone include muscles of the tongue (hyoglossus, GGM, and intrinsic muscles of the tongue), the suprahyoid muscles (digastric, stylohyoid, geniohyoid, and mylohyoid muscles) and inferiorly, the strap muscles (thyrohyoid, omohyoid, and sternohyoid muscles). The greater cornua also provide attachments to the middle constrictor muscle (**Fig. 6**). In clinical assessments of patients, the distance between the hyoid bone and the mandibular plate is commonly examined (the hyoid mandibular plane distance, H-MP). The longer length of the H-MP has been shown to correlate with OSA.[25,26] The dimensions of the hyoid bone have been studied by Ha and colleagues,[27] who retrospectively analyzed male patients, with or without OSA, by using polysomnography and axial CT images of the hyoid. The distance between the greater horns and the anteroposterior distance between the most anterior part of the body of the hyoid and the axis through the greater horns significantly correlated with the severity of OSA. Further study of this "restrictive" hyoid bone theory might be of interest in the further evaluation of expansion surgery of the hyoid or its sectioning. It is evident that the hypopharyngeal airway can decrease by almost one-third with simple postural changes, when the patient moves from the upright to the supine position.[28] In canine studies in the early 1980s, with a stainless-steel brace, it was demonstrated that anterior positioning of the hyoid body and lateral displacement of the greater cornua can expand the hypopharyngeal and tongue base airway.[29]

It is understandable that the hyoid bone and its close relationship with the hypopharynx and tongue have played an important role in the development of surgery for OSA. It can almost be likened to a convenient "handlebar" to open the pharynx and pull the tongue forward. The significance of hyoid suspension, likely through its effect

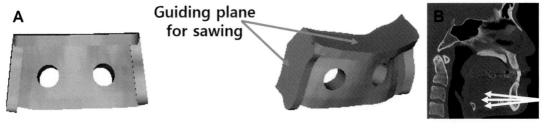

Fig. 4. Design osteotomy guide template. (*A*) Guide template in virtual simulation surgery. (*B*) Different plane of osteotomy is possible in one position of outer table like arrow. However, it is possible to perform a bone cut in correct direction after using 3-D image CT scan and guide template.

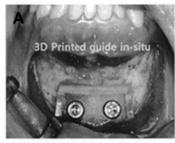 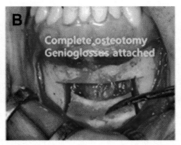 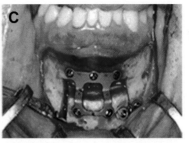

Fig. 5. Application to real surgery. During real surgery, the 3-D template prepared in this simulation process can be placed in the mandible of the patient (*A*) and guided osteotomy can be performed along the margin of the template (*B*). The advancement of bone fragments isolated from the mandible can be appropriately controlled through osteotomy by using prefabricated fixation plates and screws prepared during simulation surgery (*C*).

on the hyoglossus muscle and the intrinsic and middle constrictor muscles, was well appreciated by Riley and colleagues[30] in the early 1980s. Hyoid suspension to the lower border of the mandible by using fascia lata with the division of the infrahyoid muscles was their preferred technique. The procedure was performed as a part of multilevel airway expansion surgery, together with mandibular or maxillomandibular osteotomies and their advancement. In the early 1990s, Riley and colleagues[31] modified their technique to hyoid-thyroid-pexia, which this article refers to as "hyo-thyroidopexy." The procedure involves suturing the hyoid bone to the thyroid cartilage with partial release of the suprahyoid muscles and division of the stylohyoid ligaments attached to the lesser cornua (**Fig. 7**).

The author's (VA) preferred technique is hyo-thyroidopexy through a transverse skin crease incision placed halfway between the hyoid bone and the thyroid notch. Platysmal flaps are raised both superiorly and inferiorly, which can be retracted with stay sutures. The hyoid bone is clearly demarcated with monopolar diathermy via release of tissues and limited release of the suprahyoid muscle fibers. At our institution, the

stylohyoid muscles are not routinely divided. The superior border of the thyroid cartilage is clearly identified by dividing the sternohyoid strap muscle fibers. Our preferred sutures are Ethibond 2, V37 polyester sutures on a 40-mm taper-cut needle. Four sutures are applied through the upper thyroid cartilage, 2 on each thyroid ala. Each needle is passed deep to the hyoid; by hugging its deep surface, the tip is gently rotated through, immediately above the hyoid. All 4 sutures are passed before tying. The apposition of the hyoid and thyroid cartilage is facilitated by the surgical assistant with a pair of Littlewood tissue forceps on the body of the hyoid, displacing it caudally while gently pushing the larynx upward with the other hand. The 4 sutures can then be tied snugly (**Fig. 8**). Complications are rare; some temporary discomfort in swallowing and feeling of neck tightness may be experienced by the patient, which either settles or is adapted to over time.[32]

Other techniques of hyothyroidopexy include Hormann stainless-steel wire,[33] which sometimes cuts through the cartilage. Piccin and colleagues[34] in Italy modified the technique by using 2-mm titanium plates on the thyroid cartilage and passing the wire through the plate instead.

Hyoid expansion with an implantable device (the Air Frame system) has been examined in attempts to open the hypopharynx,[35] which did not result in significant improvements in sleep parameters. In the 1980s, Kaya[36] sectioned the hyoid bone in a Sistrunk operation in 2 patients with OSA; this was reported to yield favorable results.

It is difficult to ascertain the exact contribution of the hyoid suspension or hyothyroidopexy in a multilevel surgical procedure for OSA, as there is a lack of focused prospective randomized studies. A systematic review and meta-analysis by Song and colleagues[37] provided helpful context for the available information. In total,

Fig. 6. The hyoid bone with its muscle attachments illustrated.

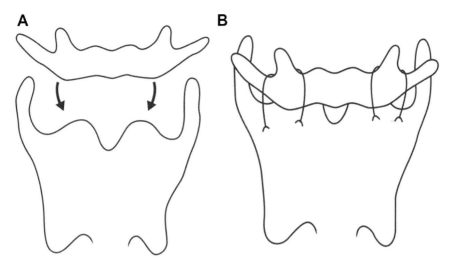

Fig. 7. Hyothyroidopexy. (*A*) The hyoid bone and thyroid cartilage are released with monopolar dissection of adjacent muscle. (*B*) Four sutures are done between hyoid bone and superior border of thyroid cartilage with Ethibond 2 suture material.

498 studies were screened and 64 were reviewed; 9 met the criteria for inclusion, with a total of 101 patients. In patients undergoing isolated hyoid surgery for OSA, hyoid suspension reduced the apnea-hypopnea index (AHI) by 38.3%, whereas for hyothyroidopexy, an AHI reduction of 50.7% was achieved. In isolated hyoid expansion, a 7.1% improvement of AHI was observed. This indicates that hyothyroidopexy is likely to contribute to the overall improvement both as a single procedure or as part of a multilevel procedure; moreover, it is likely superior to hyoid suspension, although the hyoid is typically situated at a lower level in many patients with OSA.[38] The systematic review and meta-analysis was, of course, limited by the quality of the published studies available; most were case-control or retrospective case series. In 2005, den Herder and colleagues[39] revealed that hyothyroidopexy alone as a primary procedure can achieve better results than when performed as a secondary procedure (eg, for salvage after a uvulopalatopharyngoplasty failure). The residual obstruction in secondary cases was likely to have altered the laxity of tissues and degree of tissue swelling, thus limiting the response.

Standalone primary hyoid surgery is seldom performed for patients with OSA. Likewise, hyoid surgery is often not performed alongside maxillomandibular advancement, with or without pharyngeal surgery. The effect of the likely preferred hyothyroidopexy in a multilevel procedure requires further evaluation.

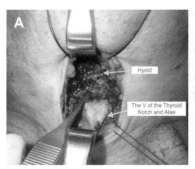
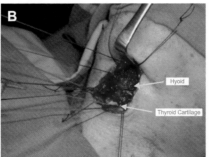
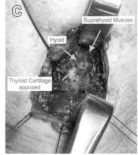

Fig. 8. Surgical procedures of the hyothyroidopexy. (*A*) Exposure via horizontal cervical skin crease incision placed midway between the hyoid and thyroid notch. (*B*) Four stitches, Ethibond 2 (Not 2/0 Ethibond), are passed through the upper edges of the thyroid cartilage and then over the body and greater cornua of the hyoid. All 4 sutures are passed before tying. (*C*) Stitches tied with apposition of the hyoid and thyroid cartilage with the help of an assistant with a pair of Littlewood forceps on the hyoid pulling it down and gently easing up the trachea and thyroid cartilage with the other hand.

REFERENCES

1. Kim AM, Keenan BT, Jackson N, et al. Tongue fat and its relationship to obstructive sleep apnea. Sleep 2014;37:1639–48.
2. Lowe AA, Gionhaku N, Takeuchi K, et al. Three-dimensional CT reconstructions of tongue and airway in adult subjects with obstructive sleep apnea. Am J Orthod Dentofacial Orthop 1986;90:364–74.
3. Lowe AA. The tongue and airway. Otolaryngol Clin North Am 1990;23:677–98.
4. Riley RW, Powell NB, Guilleminault C. Obstructive sleep apnea and the hyoid: a revised surgical procedure. Otolaryngol Head Neck Surg 1994;111:717–21.
5. Riley RW, Powell NB, Guilleminault C, et al. Maxillary-mandibular and hyoid advancement: an alternative to tracheostomy on obstructive sleep apnea. Otolaryngol Head Neck Surg 1986;94:584–8.
6. Lee NR. Genioglossus muscle advancement techniques for obstructive sleep apnea. Oral Maxillofac Surg Clin North Am 2002;14:377–84.
7. Powell N, Guilleminault C, Riley R, et al. Mandibular advancement and obstructive sleep apnea syndrome. Bull Eur Physiopathol Respir 1983;19:607–10.
8. Riley RW, Powell NB, Guilleminault C. Inferior sagittal osteotomy of the mandible with hyoid myotomy-suspension: a new procedure for obstructive sleep apnea. Otolaryngol Head Neck Surg 1986;94:589–93.
9. Riley RW, Powell NB, Guilleminault C. Obstructive sleep apnea syndrome: a review of 306 consecutively treated surgical patients. Otolaryngol Head Neck Surg 1993;108:117–25.
10. Dattilo DJ. The mandibular trapezoid osteotomy for the treatment of obstructive sleep apnea: report of a case. J Oral Maxillofac Surg 1998;56:1442–6.
11. Dattilo DJ, Aynechi M. Modification of the anterior mandibular osteotomy for genioglossus advancement with hyoid suspension for obstructive sleep apnea. J Oral Maxillofac Surg 2007;65:1876–9.
12. Miller FR, Watson D, Boseley M. The role of the Genial Bone Advancement Trephine system in conjunction with uvulopalatopharyngoplasty in the multilevel management of obstructive sleep apnea. Otolaryngol Head Neck Surg 2004;130:73–9.
13. Hendler BH, Costello BJ, Silverstein K, et al. A protocol for uvulopalatopharyngoplasty, mortised genioplasty, and maxillomandibular advancement in patients with obstructive sleep apnea: an analysis of 40 cases. J Oral Maxillofac Surg 2001;59:892–7.
14. Garcia Vega JR, de la Plata MM, Galindo N, et al. Genioglossus muscle advancement: a modification of the conventional technique. J Craniomaxillofac Surg 2014;42:239–44.
15. Li KK, Riley RW, Powell NB, et al. Obstructive sleep apnea surgery: genioglossus advancement revisited. J Oral Maxillofac Surg 2001;59:1181–4.
16. Yin SK, Yi HL, Lu WY, et al. Anatomic and spiral computed tomographic study of the genial tubercles for genioglossus advancement. Otolaryngol Head Neck Surg 2007;136:632–7.
17. Hueman EM, Noujeim ME, Langlais RP, et al. Accuracy of cone beam computed tomography in determining the location of the genial tubercle. Otolaryngol Head Neck Surg 2007;137:115–8.
18. Wang YC, Liao YF, Li HY, et al. Genial tubercle position and dimensions by cone-beam computerized tomography in a Taiwanese sample. Oral Surg Oral Med Oral Pathol Oral Radiol 2012;113:e46–50.
19. Jung SY, Shin SY, Lee KH, et al. Analysis of mandibular structure using 3D facial computed tomography. Otolaryngol Head Neck Surg 2014;151:760–4.
20. Katsumata A, Ariji Y, Langlais RP. Three dimensional computed tomography in dentistry. Dent Clin North Am 2000;44:395–410.
21. Mintz SM, Ettinger AC, Geist JR, et al. Anatomic relationship of the genial tubercles to the dentition as determined by cross-sectional tomography. J Oral Maxillofac Surg 1995;53:1324–6.
22. Jung SY, Eun YG, Min JY, et al. Anatomical analysis to establish the optimal positioning of an osteotomy for genioglossal advancement-a trial in cadavers. Br J Oral Maxillofac Surg 2018;56(8):671–7.
23. Whyms BJ, Vorperian HK, Genty LR, et al. The effect of computed tomographic scanner parameters and 3-dimensional volume rendering techniques on the accuracy of linear, angular, and volumetric measurements of the mandible. Oral Surg Oral Med Oral Pathol Oral Radiol 2013;115:682–91.
24. Lee JW, Lee DW, Ohe JY, et al. Accurate genial tubercle capturing method using computer-assisted virtual surgery for genioglossus advancement. Br J Oral Maxillofac Surg 2017;55:92–3.
25. Julià-Serdà G, Pérez-Peñate G, Saavedra-Santana P, et al. Usefulness of cephalometry in sparing polysomnography of patients with suspected obstructive sleep apnea. Sleep Breath 2006;10:181–7.
26. Barrera JE, Pau CY, Forest VI, et al. Anatomic measures of upper airway structures in obstructive sleep apnea. World J Otorhinolaryngol Head Neck Surg 2017;3:85–91.
27. Ha JG, Min HJ, Ahn SH, et al. The dimension of hyoid bone is independently associated with the severity of obstructive sleep apnea. PLoS One 2013;8:e81590.
28. Camacho M, Capasso R, Schendel S. Airway changes in obstructive sleep apnoea patients associated with a supine versus an upright position examined using cone beam computed tomography. J Laryngol Otol 2014;128:824–30.

29. Patton TJ, Thawley SE, Waters RC, et al. Expansion hyoidplasty: a potential surgical procedure designed for selected patients with obstructive sleep apnoea syndrome. Experimental canine results. Laryngoscope 1983;93:1387–96.

30. Riley R, Guilleminault C, Powell N, et al. Mandibular osteotomy and hyoid bone advancement for obstructive sleep apnea: a case report. Sleep 1984;7:79–82.

31. Riley RW, Powell NB, Guilleminault C. Obstructive sleep apnea syndrome: a surgical protocol for dynamic upper airway reconstruction. J Oral Maxillofac Surg 1993;51:742–9.

32. Richard W, Timmer F, van Tinteren H, et al. Complications of hyoid suspension in the treatment of obstructive sleep apnea syndrome. Eur Arch Otorhinolaryngol 2011;268:631–5.

33. Hormann K, Baisch A. The hyoid suspension. Laryngoscope 2004;114:1677–9.

34. Piccin O, Scaramuzzino G, Martone C, et al. Modified hyoid suspension technique in the treatment of multilevel related obstructive sleep apnea. Otolaryngol Head Neck Surg 2014;150:321–4.

35. Hamans E, Stuck BA, de Vries N, et al. Hyoid expansion as a treatment for obstructive sleep apnea: a pilot study. Sleep Breath 2013;17:195–201.

36. Kaya N. Sectioning the hyoid bone as a therapeutic approach for obstructive sleep apnea. Sleep 1984; 7:77–8.

37. Song SA, Wei JM, Buttram J, et al. Hyoid surgery alone for obstructive sleep apnea: a systematic review and meta-analysis. Laryngoscope 2016;126: 1702–8.

38. Guilleminault C, Riley R, Powell N. Obstructive sleep apnea and abnormal cephalometric measurements, implications for treatment. Chest 1984;86:793–4.

39. den Herder C, van Tinteren H, de Vries N. Hyoidthyroidpexia: a surgical treatment for sleep apnea syndrome. Laryngoscope 2005;115:740–5.

Maxillomandibular Rotational Advancement
Airway, Aesthetics, and Angle's Considerations

Clement Cheng-Hui Lin, MD, MS[a,b,c,*],
Po-fang Wang, MD[a,b,c],
Shaun Ray Han Loh, MBBS, MRCS, Mmed ORL[a,d],
Hung Tuan Lau, MBBS, MRCS, Mmed ORL[a,e],
Sam Sheng-Ping Hsu, DDS, MS[a,f,1]

KEYWORDS

- Maxillomandibular advancement • OSA • Treatment protocol • Surgical design

KEY POINTS

- Comprehensive craniofacial evaluation is essential for selection and planning of surgical treatment.
- Maxillomandibular advancement (MMA) is the most effective surgery for apnea-hypopnea index reduction.
- Surgical weight reduction and pharyngeal airway surgery are recommended for patients with obesity and tonsillar hypertrophy, respectively.
- Comprehensive cephalometry and computer-aided surgical simulation are crucial to generate a feasible surgical plan.
- With different craniofacial patterns, patients with obstructive sleep apnea need a personalized surgical plan of MMA to correct the airway, occlusion, and aethetics simultaneously.

INTRODUCTION

Maxillomandibular advancement (MMA) has been recognized as the most effective primary surgery for the treatment of obstructive sleep apnea (OSA) in terms of the reduction of apnea-hypopnea index (AHI).[1] Patients with high residual AHI or respiratory disturbance index after other surgical procedures could also benefit from MMA.[2] In long-term follow-up studies, MMA was found to be stable in both the maxillomandibular skeleton and polysomnographic outcomes. The success rate can be as high as 100% in young (<45 years old) and thin (body mass index

Disclosure: Part of this work was supported by Chang Gung Momorial Hospital, Taiwan (CRRPG5C0233)
[a] Department of Plastic and Reconstructive Surgery, Craniofacial Center, Chang Gung Memorial Hospital, No. 5, Fuxing Road, Guishan District, Taoyuan 333, Taiwan; [b] Craniofacial Research Center, Chang Gung Memorial Hospital, No. 5, Fuxing Road, Guishan District, Taoyuan 333, Taiwan; [c] School of Medicine, Chang Gung University, 259 Wenhua 1st Road, Guishan District, Taoyuan 333, Taiwan; [d] Department of Otolaryngology, Singhealth Duke-NUS Sleep Centre, Singapore General Hospital, Outram Road, Singapore 169608, Singapore; [e] Department of Otolaryngology (ENT)–Head and Neck Surgery, Khoo Teck Puat Hospital, 90 Yishun Central, Singapore 768828, Singapore; [f] Esthetic Dent Clinic, No.380, Section 4, Xinyi Road, Da'an District, Taipei 106, Taiwan
[1] Present address: 11490 6F, 187, Sec. 6, Minquan East Road, Neihu District, Taipei, Taiwan.
* Corresponding author. Department of Plastic and Reconstructive Surgery, Chang Gung Memorial Hospital, No. 5, Fuxing Road, Guishan District, Taoyuan, Taiwan.
E-mail address: clementlin0614@yahoo.com

[BMI <25]) patients with significant maxillomandibular retrognathism (angle formation by cephalometric landmarks Sella-Nasion and Nasion-point B of mandible [SNB] <75⁰).[3] The surgical success and cure rates of MMA for OSA treatment were 86.0% and 43.2%, respectively, according to a meta-analysis.[4] Long-term success of MMA was 89% by pooled data analysis from the same study.

Clinically, the modified Mallampati scale (with tongue kept in the oral cavity), tonsil size grading, and BMI are the 3 key evaluations for OSA surgery. The modified Mallampati scale shows the disproportion between soft tissue volume and the size of oral cavity. In patients with OSA and high Mallampati scale of III or IV, maxillofacial retrognathism is a common finding. In another aspect, the tonsil grading depicts the ratio of pharyngeal lateral (LAT) dimension occupied by the hypertrophic tonsils. With a high tonsil grading of III or IV, a patient with OSA has a better chance to improve by tonsillectomy with uvulopalatopharyngoplasty.[5] For patients with low tonsil grading and high Mallampati scale, MMA could be considered the first-line surgical option. Pertinently, BMI is an important and independent factor for OSA. A greater BMI can result in higher AHI in patients with equal cephalometric measurements.[6] An increase in BMI is also a main reason for relapse after all types of OSA surgery. For patients with obesity, bariatric surgery has become one treatment option to improve OSA (**Fig. 1**).

The surgical design of conventional MMA includes maxillary and mandibular osteotomies, anterior reposition of maxillomandibular complex (MMC) for more than 10 mm, and anterior inferior mandibular osteotomy (or genioglossus advancement). MMA can enlarge the maxillomandibular skeletal frame, expand the pharyngeal airway, and reinforce the genioglossus muscle tension. The conventional design may be proper for the patient with a normal facial profile. However, along with a large advancement of MMC, the facial profile may become protrusive and unacceptable to patients with maxillary protrusion and convex profile, which is commonly seen in the Asian population. During surgery, it is common for the mandible to be advanced much more than 10 mm, which is usually beyond the limit of maxillary advancement. A modification of surgical design is needed to coordinate maximal advancement in both jaws and create an optimal pharyngeal airway enlargement.

To improve the surgical design of MMA, careful consideration on the airway, the aesthetics, and the angle's classification are mandatory.

The Airway

The pharyngeal airway responds to MMA by expansion in both anteroposterior (AP) and LAT dimensions. With conventional MMA advancement of 10 mm in a 3-dimensional computed tomography (3D CT) study,[7] the AP dimension of pharyngeal airway increases, on average, 5.6 mm (56%)

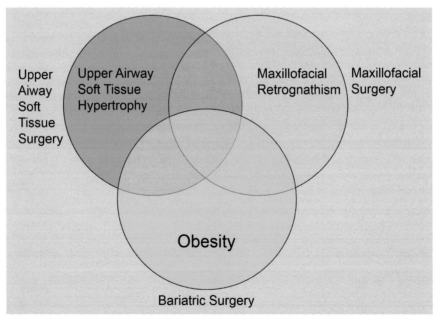

Fig. 1. Three types of surgical treatment for OSA, directing to correct 3 types of anatomic abnormalities. For patients with multiple types of deformity, multidisciplinary treatments are indicated.

of the advancement amount at the velopharynx, 4.5 mm (45%) at the retro-uvula, 4.9 mm (49%) at the oropharynx, and 5.8 mm (58%) at the retroglossal airway. Surprisingly, the LAT dimension of pharyngeal airway increases 7.1 mm (71% of advancement amount) at the velopharynx, 5.7 mm (57%) at the retro-uvula, 13.2 mm (132%) at the oropharynx, and 6.6 mm (66%) at the retroglossal airway. Skeletal advancement can dilate the LAT dimension of the pharyngeal airway more than twice that of the AP expansion. The ratio of the LAT/AP dimension increases up to 2.37 over the oropharyngeal level. However, the AP dimension has a limited increase of less than 60% of the unidirectional advancement of MMC. For patients with a narrow pharyngeal airway (<4 mm in AP dimension), the use of conventional MMA would be difficult to achieve the goal for expanding the AP pharyngeal airway space up to 10 mm.

In common occurrence, the mandible can be advanced up to 12 to 15 mm. Maintaining the maximum mandibular advancement to harness its airway expansion effect would result in a discrepancy between maxillary and mandibular advancement, which may create negative overjet and consequent malocclusion. In order to correct the negative overjet, counterclockwise rotation of both maxillary and mandibular segments is a crucial step. With counterclockwise rotational advancement, the mandible can be advanced much more than the maxilla, and normal occlusion can be maintained at the same time (**Fig. 2**). After counterclockwise rotational advancement, the pharyngeal airway has 47% and 76% (of the amount of mandibular advancement) increase in AP dimension at the velopharynx and retroglossal area, respectively.[8]

In Taiwan, segmental osteotomies are included in the surgical plan of MMA. Combined with counterclockwise rotation, segmental Le Fort I maxillary osteotomy can further advance the posterior nasal spine and palatine bone by 7 mm, provided by alveolar bone reduction after extraction or edentulous spaces. By segmental maxillomandibular rotational advancement (SMMRA), the pharyngeal airway can be increased in AP dimension of the velopharynx by 60% (of the amount of mandibular advancement), and 70% (of the mandibular advancement) at the oropharynx.[9]

In consideration of the airway, all parts of the maxillomandibular skeleton need to be advanced as much as possible. After Le Fort I maxillary and bilateral sagittal splits mandibular osteotomies, the limits on advancement of upper and lower jaws are defined by the neurovascular bundles of the greater palatine nerve and vessels to the posterior maxilla, and the mandibular nerve and vessels to the mandible. By integrating counterclockwise rotation of the maxilla, mandible, and the occlusal plane into the surgical design, the MMC can achieve optimal advancement in both jaws without compromising the occlusion. When necessary, segmental osteotomies can be applied to the posterior maxilla to further advance the posterior border, stretch the soft palate, and reposition it more anteriorly to enlarge the AP dimension of the velopharyngeal airway (**Fig. 3**).

The Aesthetics

Along with a large advancement in the maxillomandibular region, the dramatic changes in facial appearance have drawn significant attention from both patients and surgeons. In a

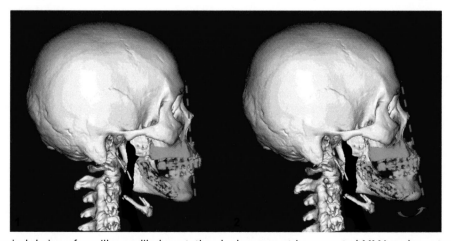

Fig. 2. Surgical design of maxillomandibular rotational advancement incorporated MMA and counterclockwise rotation, pivoted on the skeletal landmark Nasion, maintaining the angular measurement ANB, which represents the relationship between cranium, maxilla, and mandible. The facial plane is maintained normal after maxillomandibular counterclockwise rotational advancement (dashed line).

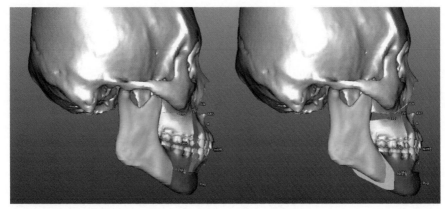

Fig. 3. Surgical design of SMMRA incorporated segmental osteotomies of maxilla and mandible to improve the bimaxillary protrusion, MMA, and counterclockwise rotation, to enlarge the oral cavity and expand the pharyngeal airway. All the skeletal landmarks move forward and/or downward.

questionnaire evaluation, most of the MMA patients subjectively experienced moderate changes of facial appearance. However, more than 90% of patients still gave positive or neutral feedback on the facial changes.[10]

From a cephalometric evaluation, Asian patients were found to have a more protrusive facial pattern and a narrower cranial base angle than Caucasian patients.[11] With conventional MMA, which advances the maxilla and mandible by the same large distance, the angular measurement of SNA (angle formation by cephalometric landmarks Sella-Nasion and Nasion-point A of maxilla) may increase more than the angular measurement of SNB. Subsequently, the measurement of ANB (the angle formed by cephalometric landmarks point A-Sella-point B) increases and makes the convex facial profile even more convex. To solve this issue, 3 different ways have been adopted in the surgical design.

Segmental osteotomy of maxilla and/or mandible

The protrusive appearance of perioral soft tissue comes from the strong support by the front teeth of the upper and lower jaws. By segmental osteotomy of the maxilla (Wassmund procedure) and mandible (Köle procedure), the proclination of front teeth can be reduced through pitch rotation of anterior segments, and the protrusive appearance can thus be improved.[12] Modified MMA using maxillomandibular segmental osteotomies has been shown to effectively treat OSA whilst maintaining an acceptable facial profile at the same time.[13] Contrary to the backward rotation of anterior segments in aesthetic orthognathic surgery, it has been emphasized that all the dentoskeletal segments should be moved forward

to ensure the enlargement of the maxillofacial frame and oral cavity on patients with OSA.[9]

Counterclockwise rotation of maxillomandibular advancement

Incorporation of counterclockwise rotation of the MMC in the surgical planning of MMA can help maintain the facial relationship between cranium, midface (the maxilla), and lower face (the mandible). The ANB angle is the key to achieve a normal facial relationship. By moving the MMC, rotational forward, pivoted on the facial skeletal landmark N (Nasion), the ANB angle can be kept within normal range. Especially for patients with OSA and maxillomandibular retrusion, the deformity with a high occlusal plane angle and a high mandibular plane angle is commonly seen. Counterclockwise rotation of MMC can improve the occlusal plane and mandibular plane angle while maintaining the facial relationship[9] (see **Fig. 2**).

Genioplasty

Chin retrusion with flat labiomental curve is a frequent combination in patients with mandibular retrusion. To improve the labiomental fold and chin projection, a sliding genioplasty can be performed as a horizontal osteotomy over the central portion of the mandible lower than bilateral mental nerve, and advancing the bony segment forward to enhance the chin projection. In patients with OSA, the surgical design of genioplasty can be modified to cut more superiorly at the central area below the lower central incisors and to include the genioglossus tubercle within the advancing segment. The additional advancement of the genioglossus tubercle can help to increase the tension of the genioglossus and geniohyoid muscles, pull the tongue forward, and indirectly suspend the hyoid. According to different design

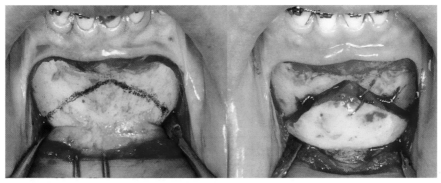

Fig. 4. Triangular genioplasty, including genioglossus tubercle advancement, to augment chin contour and increase tension of genioglossus and geniohyoid at the same time.

descriptions in the literature, the genioplasty can be designed as trapezoid, mortise, or triangular shapes[14] (**Fig. 4**).

The Angle's Classification

Although class II malocclusion can be observed in most patients with OSA, not everyone with class I or class III occlusion is exempt from the disorder. Therefore sleep surgeons require various strategies to build up tailored surgical plans suitable for patients with OSA of different facial patterns (**Table 1**). A comprehensive cephalometric evaluation is mandatory for the surgical planning. Cone-beam CT examination provides 3D images for cephalometric, airway measurements, and surgical simulation when applied to a 3D surgical planning program.

Class I

Patients with class I occlusion have normal cephalometry and a narrow airway. An appropriate surgical option would be MMA combined with counterclockwise rotation pivoting on the Nasion. With this design, the normal ANB angle can be maintained. The AP dimension of the maxillofacial region would be enlarged without changing the angular relationship among cranium, maxilla, and mandible. Both airway and aethetic considerations are satisfied, and the occlusal relationship is maintained as class I.

Class II

Patients with OSA with class II malocclusion have mandibular retrognathism, large overjet, and/or a high mandibular plane angle. With the surgical design to correct class II malocclusion, the mandible may be advanced by the amount of abnormal overjet. In order to further expand the pharyngeal airway, the MMC needs to be advanced to the maximal extent of the mandible. For patients with bimaxillary protrusion, segmental osteotomies of the maxilla (Wassmund procedure) and/or the mandible (Köle procedure) can be used to reduce the proclination of upper and lower front teeth. Segmental osteotomy of the maxilla can also further advance the posterior border of the maxilla, pull the soft palate forward, thus enlarging the velopharynx. Genioplasty, including the genioglossus tubercle, can increase the tension of genioglossus and geniohyoid muscles and help maintain the retroglossal airway dimension.[9]

Class III

In patients with OSA with class III malocclusion, a narrow velopharyngeal airway is a common situation due to maxillary hypoplasia and retrusion. High and narrow maxilla with restricted nasal passages can also exist. Maxillary advancement is essential to correct class III malocclusion and enlarge the velopharynx. Maxillary expansion is indicated in patients with high nasal resistance. When a narrow retroglossal airway is noted, mandibular advancement with counterclockwise rotation may be necessary to expand the airway and fix the occlusion at the same time.

Table 1	
Surgical design of maxillomandibular advancement for patients with obstructive sleep apnea with various facial patterns	
Class	**Surgical Design**
I	MMA ± counterclockwise rotation
II	SMMRA + genioplasty
III	Maxillomandibular rotational advancement

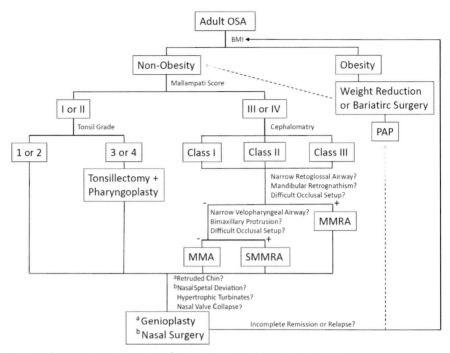

Fig. 5. Algorithm of surgical considerations for OSA. PAP, positive airway pressure.

SUMMARY

The success of surgical treatment of adult patients with OSA relies on accurate differential diagnosis by clinical history, physical examination of craniofacial structures, and standard overnight polysomnography. To have the best effectiveness, the surgical options need to be directed to the anatomic abnormality related to the pathophysiology of OSA.

Obesity has an independent negative impact on the soft tissue of the pharyngeal airway and the effectiveness of surgery. A combination of positive airway pressure treatment and weight reduction, be it surgical or nonsurgical, would be the treatment of choice for patients with OSA with high BMI.

Intrapharyngeal surgery would achieve a high success rate on patients with high tonsil grading and low Mallampati scale, representing a strong soft tissue factor and minimal maxillofacial retrognathism. Extrapharyngeal procedures such as septoplasty and trubinate reduction may be performed as an adjunctive procedure to improve nasal patency and reduce upper airway resistance.

MMA can be the primary treatment option for nonobese patients with Mallampati scale of III or above. Cephalometry by 2-dimensional cephalogram or 3D CT images is recommended. Through comparison of cephalometric data with normative values of general population, the surgical plan can be made to meet the requirement of airway, aesthetics, and the angle's normal occlusion (**Fig. 5**).

REFERENCES

1. Prinsell JR. Primary and secondary telegnathic maxillomandibular advancement, with or without adjunctive procedures, for obstructive sleep apnea in adults: a literature review and treatment recommendations [review]. J Oral Maxillofac Surg 2012;70(7): 1659–77.

2. Zagi S, Holty JE, Certal V, et al. Maxillomandibular advancement for treatment of obstructive sleep apnea: a meta-analysis. JAMA Otolaryngol Head Neck Surg 2016;142(1):58–66.

3. Vigneron A, Tamisier R, Orset E, et al. Maxillomandibular advancement for obstructive sleep apnea syndrome treatment: long-term results. J Craniomaxillofac Surg 2017;45(2):183–91.

4. Holty JE, Guilleminault C. Maxillomandibular advancement for the treatment of obstructive sleep apnea: a systemic review and meta-analysis [reveiw]. Sleep Med Rev 2010;14(5):287–97.

5. Friedman M, Ibrahim H, Bass L. Clinical staging for sleep-disordered breathing. Otolaryngol Head Neck Surg 2002;127(1):13–21.

6. Partinen M, Guilleminault C, Quera-Salva MA, et al. Obstructive sleep apnea and cephalometric roentgenograms. The role of anatomic upper airway abnormalities in the definition of abnormal

breathing during sleep. Chest 1988;93(6): 1199–205.

7. Fairburn SC, Waite PD, Vilos G, et al. Three-dimensional changes in upper airways of patients with obstructive sleep apnea following maxillomandibular advancement. J Oral Maxillofac Surg 2007; 65(1):6–12.

8. Mehra P, Downie M, Pita MC, et al. Pharyngeal airway space changes after counterclockwise rotation of the maxillomandibular complex. Am J Orthod Dentofacial Orthop 2001;120(2):154–9.

9. Lin CH, Liao YF, Chen NH, et al. Three-dimensional computed tomography in obstructive sleep apneics treated by maxillomandibular advancement. Laryngoscope 2011;121(6):1336–47.

10. Li KK, Riley RW, Powell NB, et al. Patient's perception of the facial appearance after maxillomandibular advancement for obstructive sleep apne syndrome. J Oral Maxillofac Surg 2001;59(4):377–80 [discussion: 380–1].

11. Li KK, Powell NB, Kushida C, et al. A comparison of Asian and white patients with obstructive sleep apnea syndrome. Laryngoscope 1999;109(12):1937–40.

12. Chu YM, Chen P-HR, Morris DE, et al. Surgical approach to the patient with bimaxillary protrusion. Clin Plast Surg 2007;34(3):535–46.

13. Goh YH, Lim KA. Modified maxillomandibular advancement for the treatment of obstructive sleep apnea: a preliminary report. Laryngoscope 2003; 113:1577–82.

14. Singhal D, Hsu SS, Lin CH, et al. Trapezoid mortised genioplasty: a further refinement of mortised genioplasty. Laryngoscope 2013;123(10):2578–82.

Addressing the Tone and Synchrony Issue During Sleep: Pacing the Hypoglossal Nerve

Clemens Heiser, MD*, Benedikt Hofauer, MD

KEYWORDS

- Obstructive sleep apnea • Hypoglossal nerve stimulation • Upper airway stimulation
- Cross motor innervation • Hypoglossal nerve

KEY POINTS

- Upper airway stimulation enables an effective and sustained reduction of the severity of obstructive sleep apnea.
- Upper airway stimulation reduces the subjective daytime sleepiness in patients with obstructive sleep apnea.
- The amount of light sleep can be reduced with upper airway stimulation.
- Patients use upper airway stimulation with a high adherence.
- Upper airway stimulation has a higher responder rate than uvulopalatopharyngoplasty and expansion sphincter pharyngoplasty in comparable patient cohorts.

INTRODUCTION

Obstructive sleep apnea (OSA) is the most common sleep-disordered breathing disorder and is characterized by recurrent narrowing and obstruction of the upper respiratory tract, which results in intermittent drops of oxygen saturation, activation of the sympathetic nervous system, and consequently, increased sleep fragmentation as well as reduction of deep and rapid eye movement (REM) sleep. This sleep fragmentation causes on the one hand morning and daytime sleepiness and thus a reduction of quality of life; on the other hand, it is now also known that patients with untreated OSA are at a higher risk for cardiovascular diseases (eg, arterial hypertension, coronary heart disease, stroke), but also metabolic diseases (eg, diabetes mellitus).[1,2]

During the last few years, upper airway stimulation (UAS) became widely available as an alternative treatment option for patients with OSA, who have proven to be nonadherent to continuous positive airway pressure therapy. The effect on the upper airways is generated by the stimulation of the hypoglossal nerve, which can either be achieved by a breath-synchronized (Inspire II/IV System, Inspire Medical Systems, Maple Grove, MN, USA) or a continuous stimulation (ImThera aura, 6000 system, LivaNova, London, United Kingdom).[3–5] Further stimulation systems are currently under development, such as a bilateral stimulations system, for the most distal fibers of the hypoglossal nerve with an implantable stimulator, which receives energy pulses from an external patch (Nyxoah SAT System, Nyxoah, Mont-St-Guibert, Belgium).

In this article, studies on various aspects of UAS addressing different aspects of this novel therapy are presented in an educational review. Because of the so far only small number of studies published on the continuous nightly stimulation of the hypoglossal nerve, the main focus of this article is on the breath-synchronized stimulation.

Disclosure Statement: Dr Heiser is a consultant for Inspire Medical Systems and received research grants from Inspire Medical Systems. Dr Hofauer received travel expenses and honoraria from Inspire Medical Systems.
Department of Otorhinolaryngology, Head and Neck Surgery, Klinikum Rechts der Isar, Technische Universitat Munchen, Ismaninger Street. 22, Munich 81675, Germany
* Corresponding author.
E-mail address: hno@heiser-online.com

Sleep Med Clin 14 (2019) 91–97
https://doi.org/10.1016/j.jsmc.2018.10.010
1556-407X/19/© 2018 Elsevier Inc. All rights reserved.

TREATMENT OF THE DISORDERED BREATHING

The effect of the breath-synchronized UAS on the apnea hypopnea index (AHI) and the oxygen desaturation index (ODI) was first impressively demonstrated in an international multicentric study (STAR study, Stimulation Therapy for Apnea Reduction) and published in 2014.[3] Within a collective of 126 patients with moderate to severe OSA, it was shown that preoperative AHI with an average of 32.0/h could be decreased to an average of 15.3/h after 12 months (P<.001), and the preoperative ODI of 28.9/h down to 13.9/h (P<.001).[3] In this patient population, a success rate, according to the Sher criteria (reduction of AHI of more than 50% and AHI <20/h), of 66% was achieved. Within this collective, the effect of the UAS has been further monitored with results already published for the time points 18, 24, 36, and 48 months after the implantation.[6–9] With a reduction of the original AHI value to an average of 11.5/h after 3 years, a lasting effect of the therapy was observed.[2,7] Recently, the 5-year outcomes of the STAR trial were published. Seventy-one of the originally included patients conducted a voluntary polysomnography 60 months after the implantation, and a stable reduction of AHI and ODI compared with the 12- and 36-month assessment was observed with a responder rate according to Sher of 75%.[10]

Within the STAR trial, the first 46 successfully treated patients were randomized to either therapy maintenance or therapy withdrawal. In the withdrawal group, the therapy was stopped for 1 week 12 months after the implantation, whereas the therapy in the comparison group remained active. After 1 week, a polysomnography was performed in both groups that could show that switching off the therapy led to an increase in both AHI and ODI up to the level of the baseline values, whereas stably reduced values were shown in the maintenance group. Thereafter, the therapy was activated again for both groups, and a new polysomnography was carried out after 18 months. Here again a significant reduction of AHI and ODI was shown in both groups.[11]

A postmarket study was conducted by 3 German implantation centers (Departements of Otorhinolaryngology and Head and Neck Surgery in Mannheim, Munich and Luebeck) after the launch of the therapy. The primary aim of this project was to investigate the efficacy and safety of the UAS within another collective outside a study setting but within the clinical routine.[12,13] Sixty patients with an initial AHI of 31.2/h and an initial ODI of 27.6/h were enrolled. The AHI was reduced to an average value of 12.0/h after 6 months and 13.8/h (each P<.05) after 12 months, whereas the ODI decreased after 6 months to a value of 13.5/h and after 12 months to a value of 13.7/h (each P<.05). Separately, the monocentric experience of the Otorhinolaryngology/Head and Neck Surgery of the Klinikum Rechts der Isar (Technical University of Munich) was published.[14] Here the effect of the stimulation therapy could be confirmed. Munich was further the first stimulation center with 100 implantations in Europe (**Fig. 1, Table 1**).[2] In a subanalysis of older patients (>64 years) with UAS, again a significant reduction of both the AHI and the ODI was observed with older patients showing even higher usage of the therapy than younger patients.[15]

In a study on the effectiveness of the continuous nocturnal stimulation of the hypoglossal nerve within a collective of 46 patients, the AHI was reduced in 43 patients from a baseline of 34.9/h to 25.4/h (P = .004) after 6 months, which corresponds to a success rate of 39.5% according to the Sher criteria.[4]

REDUCTION OF SUBJECTIVE DAYTIME SLEEPINESS

The subjective level of sleepiness is evaluated by using the Epworth Sleepiness Scale (ESS) and the daytime functioning by using the Functional Outcome of Sleep Questionnaire (FOSQ). These parameters were used as secondary endpoints in the STAR study.[3] Before implantation, the ESS baseline score was 11.6 points in this patient population, assuming a pathologic level of sleepiness at 10 points and above, and a baseline FOSQ score of 14.3 (normal value should be above 17.9). During the STAR study, the ESS value was lowered to a value of 7.0 after 12 months (P<.001), and the value of the FOSQ was increased to 17.3 (P<.001), with an increase of at least 2 points reported to be clinically relevant.[3] In the most recent 5-year outcomes of the STAR trial, both the ESS and FOSQ improvements persisted during the last follow-up. The percentage of patients with a normal ESS score increased from 33% at baseline to 78%, and the percentage of patients with a normal FOSQ increased from 15% at baseline to 67% after 5 years.[10] The effect on the daytime alertness, measured by the maintenance of wakefulness test (MWT), has been evaluated recently.[16] The objective level of alertness improved from an initial MWT latency of 25.0 minutes before implantation to 36.8 minutes after 6 months (P = .006).[16]

The effect on the subjective sleepiness was also observed in context of the German postmarket study. A reduction of the subjective sleepiness from an initial ESS score of 12.8 to a value of 6.5

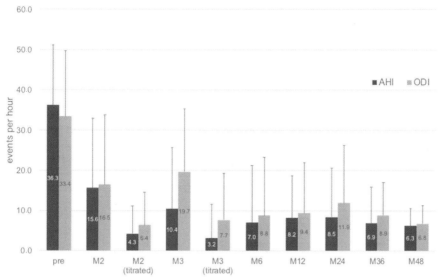

Fig. 1. AHI and ODI score at before surgery (pre), 2, 3, 6, 12, 24, 36, and 48 months after surgery (M2, M3, M6, M12, M24, M36, and M48). "M2 complete" and "M3 complete" represent the AHI score for the complete titration polysomnography (that means including the periods of insufficient stimulation). "M2 titrated" and "M3 titrated" illustrate the AHI score during the period of optimal stimulation during the polysomnography. The baseline AHI was reduced significantly to all postimplantation visits (P<.001 each). M, month.

after 12 months and an increase of the FOSQ from 13.7 at baseline to 17.5 were found.[12,13]

In the monocentric results of the Otorhinolaryngology/Head and Neck Surgery of the Klinikum Rechts der Isar, the initial ESS value of 12.6 before implantation was reduced to a value of 8.6 after 6 months and 5.9 after 12 months (P<.001).[14] Again, in the largest so far published monocentric cohort, the effect on the subjective sequela of OSA could be confirmed. **Table 2** shows a list of the main publications in the last recent years in selective UAS. An average AHI reduction of almost 80% and responder rate between 80% and 90% could be achieved in several independent trials at different centers in the world (see **Table 2**).

Table 1	
Patients' characteristics	
Characteristics	**Mean**
Age (y)	57.0 (12.0)
Sex (male/female)	89/11
BMI (kg/m^2)	29.5 (4.1)
Time difference between diagnosis of OSA and implantation (mo)	33.6 (45.1)
AHI (n/h)	36.5 (14.7)
ODI (n/h)	35.8 (16.3)
ESS	11.5 (5.3)

Table 1 shows the patient's characteristics of 100 patients with selective UAS. Data are presented as mean with standard deviation in parentheses.
Abbreviation: BMI, body mass index.

In the study of the effect of continuous stimulation of the Nervus hypoglossus, a reduction of the ESS from 12.0 before implantation to 8.3 at 6 months was observed.[4]

SLEEP STAGES AND CHARACTERISTICS

The effect of UAS on sleep architecture was investigated in a separate publication.[17] In a group of 26 patients, preoperative polysomnography showed a percentage of N1 sleep of 23.2%, N2 sleep of 57.7%, N3 sleep of 9.2%, and REM sleep of 9.5%. During the polysomnography 2 months after the implantation, a reduction of N1 sleep to 16.4% (P = .067) and a significant increase of REM sleep to 15.7% (P = .01) were observed. The latter was interpreted as an REM rebound, as a further control polysomnography revealed a slight decrease in the REM content after another month (13.5%). The reduction of the N1 sleep however was further decreased to 16.0% compared with baseline (P = .007). Similar observations have been made by Philip and colleagues.[16] Within a collective of 10 patients, again a decrease in the amount of N1 sleep was observed 6 months after the implantation compared with baseline (11.8% vs 4.2%, P = .04), whereas the amount of N2, N3, and REM sleep did not change significantly. A significant reduction of both the number of changes to wake and the sleep stage changes (11.1 vs 5.0, P<.001 and 52.7 vs 28.5, P = .007, respectively) were observed 3 months after the implantation, whereas Philip and colleagues[16] observed a trend

Table 2
Overview over the publications on selective upper airway stimulation

	Study	Year	Number of Patients	AHI-Baseline	AHI (6–12 mo)	Responders (Sher)
STAR- trial	12 mo (1 y)[3]	2014	126	29.3 ± 11.8	8.7 ± 16.1	66%
	12 mo (withdrawl study)[11]	2014	46	31.3 ± 12.3	7.2 ± 5.0	n.a.
				30.1 ± 11.4	25.8 ± 16.2	n.a.
	18 mo (1.5 y)[9]	2015	126	29.3 ± 11.8	9.7 ± 14.0	66%
	36 mo (3 y)[7]	2015	116	28.2 ± 14.0	6.0 ± 14.0	74%
	60 mo (5 y)[10]	2018	97	29.3 ± 11.8	6.2 ± 16.3	75%
German Post-Market Study	6 mo[13]	2016	60	28.6 ± 13.2	8.3 ± 14.8	68%
	12 mo (1 y)[12]	2017	60	28.6 ± 13.2	9.5 ± 14.8	82%
Single Center	Munich[14]	2016	30	32.9 ± 11.2	7.1 ± 5.9	97%
	Pittsburgh[33]	2016	20	33.3 ± 13.0	5.1 ± 4.3	95%
	Cleveland (UPPP vs UAS)[18]	2018	20 (UAS)	38.9 ± 12.5	4.5 ± 4.8	100%
			20 (UPPP)	40.3 ± 12.4	28.8 ± 25.4	40%
	Philadelphia & Pittsburgh[34]	2017	48 (Phil)	35.8 ± 20.8	6.3 ± 11.5	91%
			49 (Pitt)	35.2 ± 15.3	6.2 ± 6.1	91%
	Philadelphia[19]	2018	49	39.3 ± 2.7	3.9 ± 1.2	96%
Others	Elderly Patients[15]	2018	31 (>65 y)	28.7 ± 13.0	6.0 ± 14.6	81%
			31 (<65 y)	28.4 ± 10.6	6.0 ± 6.9	84%
ADHERE (6–12 mo; on going)[35]		2018	301	35.6 ± 15.3	10.2 ± 12.9	78%
			508	34.0 ± 15.7	7.0 ± 13.3	81%

Abbreviations: ADHERE, Adherence and Outcome for Upper Airway Stimulation for OSA International Registry; n.a., not applicable; Phil, Philadelphia; Pitt, Pittsburgh.

toward a reduction of the wake after sleep onset duration from 71.4 minutes at baseline to 53.4 minutes after 6 months ($P = .06$).

Further analysis of the arousal parameters showed that the total number of arousals and consequently also the arousal index decreased during this observation interval. Although the respiratory effort-dependent arousals also decreased significantly during therapy, this effect could not be observed in the movement-dependent arousals. The effect on the number of sleep stage changes, change to awake, and the exact values of the changes are as indicated in **Table 2**. This information is relevant because it has been shown that nocturnal stimulation therapy induces no sensory stimuli, which in turn could generate arousals and thus disturb the sleep architecture.

EFFECT OF UPPER AIRWAY STIMULATION COMPARED WITH ANATOMY-ALTERING SURGICAL PROCEDURES

UAS, as a surgical, not anatomy-altering but rather functional treatment, has been compared with the effect of established, anatomy-altering surgical procedures, such as uvulopalatopharyngoplasty (UPPP) or expansion sphincter pharyngoplasty (ESP). Shah and colleagues[18] compared the effect of UAS and UPPP in groups of 20 patients each with OSA. The baseline AHI in the UPPP group was 40.3/h and in the UAS group was 38.9/h. The postoperative sleep study was performed mainly after 3 to 6 months and revealed an AHI of 28.8/h ($P = .02$) in the UPPP group and 4.5/h ($P<.001$) in the UAS group. Although only 8/20 patients in the UPPP group were successfully treated according to the Sher criteria, all patients in the UAS group (20/20) responded to the therapy according to these criteria. Huntley and colleagues[19] compared the efficacy of UAS to ESP. The ESP group consisted of 33 patients with a baseline AHI of 26.7/h, and the UAS group consisted of 75 patients with a baseline AHI of 36.8/h ($P = .003$). In the postoperative sleep study, the patients in the ESP group presented with an AHI of 13.5/h and in the UAS group presented with 7.3/h ($P = .003$ between the both postoperative results). Applying the Sher criteria for the evaluation of surgical success, 63.6% in the ESP group and 86.7% in the UAS group reached this goal.

PATIENTS' EXPERIENCE WITH UPPER AIRWAY STIMULATION

The adherence to the UAS was further investigated because the therapy must be activated by the patient with a remote control every time before usage, which is a difference from the classical surgical treatment options of OSA so far, which did not require further compliance because the anatomic changes were permanent. A collective of 102 patients was investigated, which revealed a usage of 5.7 hours per night with their UAS system. Of the patients, 74.5% used the therapy more than 4 hours per night and 50% of the patients used the therapy even more than 6 hours per night.[20] The evaluation of the patients' attitude toward UAS resulted in strong agreement toward the statement "UAS reduces the problems caused by my sleep apnea." In further evaluations, information on the subjective sensation and usage habits could be gathered, which are helpful for the further consultation of potential candidates.[21] This aspect was additionally evaluated within the multicenter German postmarket study. Here a strong correlation between the postoperative AHI results and the personal satisfaction of the patients after implantation was found. Therapy usage was higher the more the patients benefited from UAS according to their self-reported outcome.[22] The impact of the hypoglossal nerve stimulation on swallowing and voice was evaluated within a prospective cohort study by application of the Voice Handicap Index-10 and Eating Assessment Tool-10 at baseline and repeatedly during 6 months after implantation. No sustained changes in voice or swallowing function were observed during the observation period.[23]

MECHANISM OF STIMULATION

The influence of the type of tongue movement on the therapeutic effect seems to have an impact on the effectiveness of UAS. In a paper on different types of tongue movement published in 2015, 3 different patterns were initially identified: bilateral protrusion, right-sided protrusion, and mixed activation. The effect of the therapy was compared between these groups, and it could be shown that patients with a mixed activation responded less well to the therapy (lower reduction of the preoperative AHI value) than the patients with a bilateral or right-sided protrusion. This observation was explained by the placement of the stimulation cuff, and the recommendation was given to place it distal enough with inclusion of the medial fibers for the innervation of the genioglossus muscle and the intrinsic musculature.[2,24–26] The stimulation cuff enables different electrode configurations. In a further work, the influence of different electrode configurations on the tongue movement was investigated. Here, it was found that the type of tongue movement can change depending on the configuration, and mostly (in 73.5% of cases) a change between a bilateral and a right-sided protrusion could be generated. Here, it was also recommended that different electrode configurations should be tested intraoperatively and that the configuration of the cuff should be controlled and, if necessary, changed during a configuration-dependent transition to a mixed activation.[2,27]

Further investigation on the effect of the stimulation of the hypoglossal nerve on the soft palate, an effect called "palatoglossus coupling," has been under further investigation. It could be shown that a bilateral protrusion is the most favorable pattern of tongue movement with the best opening of soft palate. It is therefore postulated that the stimulation of the hypoglossal nerve can also be used effectively in patients with OSA and isolated soft palate obstruction.[28]

FURTHER DEVELOPMENT OF THE OPERATIVE TECHNIQUE

With increasing experience, the surgical technique could be further optimized, such as a modified incision to visualize the hypoglossal nerve. **Fig. 2** shows a schematic drawing of the incision lines for selective UAS. A new surgical approach was developed to allow easy access to the terminating branches of the hypoglossal nerve.[29] In addition, a detailed list of surgical recommendations in special situations, such as implantation in women after breast augmentation or mastectomy, left-sided implantation, or use of UAS in patients with pacemakers, was published.[30]

With the increasing impact of this novel therapy, the anatomy of the hypoglossal nerve came into

focus. It became more relevant for surgeons to be aware of the single nerve fibers at the area of the distal nerve where the cuff is placed and to know the variations of the nerve. With the help of intraoperative documentation, a classification system could be created. Special variations of the course of the nerve were identified that are challenging for an optimal placement of the stimulation cuff.[31] This classification is intended to help surgeons to identify the individual nerve fibers and facilitate the placement of the stimulation cuff in the future. This classification is intended to help surgeons to identify the individual nerve fibers and facilitate the placement of the stimulation cuff in the future, which was further confirmed in a separate study on the use of intraoperative neuromonitoring.[32]

SUMMARY

In recent years, the evidence for the breath-synchronized UAS therapy in the treatment of OSA has steadily increased. In addition to a persistent effect on the severity of OSA, several studies have shown the positive effect of the therapy on the subjective daytime impairment of the patients. Studies on sleep architecture revealed a decrease in N1 levels during therapy and evidence of an REM rebound. With an average usage of 5.7 hours per night, a good adherence was observed. Information on the patients' experience of the stimulation therapy could be gained and used for the counseling of potential candidates for UAS. Comparisons between UAS therapy and classical surgical treatment options in OSA, such as UPPP and ESP, revealed a higher responder rate in UAS. The surgical technique could be further optimized, and recommendation for special situations during the stimulation could be shared.

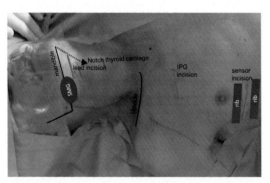

Fig. 2. The incision lines for implanting a device for selective UAS. Three incisions are needed: (1) one finger down below the mandible for the stimulation lead (stay before the anterior border of the SMG to avoid hurting the marginal mandibular nerve); (2) 3 fingers below the clavicle for the IPG; (3) between the ribs in the third to sixth intercostal space for the sensing leas. IPG, implantable pulse generator; SMG, submandibular gland.

REFERENCES

1. Strollo PJ, Rogers RM. Obstructive sleep apnea. N Engl J Med 1996;334(2):99–104.
2. Hofauer B, Heiser C. Der Einsatz der Stimulationstherapie der oberen Atemwege in Deutschland. Somnologie 2018;22:98–105.
3. Strollo PJ, Soose RJ, Maurer JT, et al. Upper-airway stimulation for obstructive sleep apnea. N Engl J Med 2014;370(2):139–49.
4. Friedman M, Jacobowitz O, Hwang MS, et al. Targeted hypoglossal nerve stimulation for the treatment of obstructive sleep apnea: six-month results. Laryngoscope 2016;126(11):2618–23.
5. Heiser C, Hofauer B. Hypoglossal nerve stimulation in patients with CPAP failure : Evolution of an alternative treatment for patients with obstructive sleep apnea. HNO 2017;65(2):99–106 [in German].

6. Soose RJ, Woodson BT, Gillespie MB, et al. Upper airway stimulation for obstructive sleep apnea: self-reported outcomes at 24 months. J Clin Sleep Med 2016;12(1):43–8.

7. Woodson BT, Soose RJ, Gillespie MB, et al. Three-year outcomes of cranial nerve stimulation for obstructive sleep apnea: the STAR trial. Otolaryngol Head Neck Surg 2016;154(1):181–8.

8. Gillespie MB, Soose RJ, Woodson BT, et al. Upper airway stimulation for obstructive sleep apnea: patient-reported outcomes after 48 months of follow-up. Otolaryngol Head Neck Surg 2017;156(4):765–71.

9. Strollo PJ, Gillespie MB, Soose RJ, et al. Upper airway stimulation for obstructive sleep apnea: durability of the treatment effect at 18 months. Sleep 2015;38(10):1593–8.

10. Woodson BT, Strohl KP, Soose RJ, et al. Upper airway stimulation for obstructive sleep apnea: 5-year outcomes. Otolaryngol Head Neck Surg 2018;159(1):194–202.

11. Woodson BT, Gillespie MB, Soose RJ, et al. Randomized controlled withdrawal study of upper airway stimulation on OSA: short- and long-term effect. Otolaryngol Head Neck Surg 2014;151(5):880–7.

12. Steffen A, Sommer JU, Hofauer B, et al. Outcome after one year of upper airway stimulation for obstructive sleep apnea in a multicenter German post-market study. Laryngoscope 2018;128(2):509–15.

13. Heiser C, Maurer JT, Hofauer B, et al. Outcomes of upper airway stimulation for obstructive sleep apnea in a multicenter German postmarket study. Otolaryngol Head Neck Surg 2017;156(2):378–84.

14. Heiser C, Knopf A, Bas M, et al. Selective upper airway stimulation for obstructive sleep apnea: a single center clinical experience. Eur Arch Otorhinolaryngol 2017;274(3):1727–34.

15. Zhu Z, Hofauer B, Wirth M, et al. Selective upper airway stimulation in older patients. Respir Med 2018;140:77–81.

16. Philip P, Heiser C, Bioulac S, et al. Hypoglossal nerve stimulation on sleep and level of alertness in OSA: a preliminary study. Neurology 2018;91(7):e615–9.

17. Hofauer B, Philip P, Wirth M, et al. Effects of upper-airway stimulation on sleep architecture in patients with obstructive sleep apnea. Sleep Breath 2017;21(4):901–8.

18. Shah J, Russell JO, Waters T, et al. Uvulopalatopharyngoplasty vs CN XII stimulation for treatment of obstructive sleep apnea: a single institution experience. Am J Otolaryngol 2018;39(3):266–70.

19. Huntley C, Chou DW, Doghramji K, et al. Comparing upper airway stimulation to expansion sphincter pharyngoplasty: a single university experience. Ann Otol Rhinol Laryngol 2018;127(6):379–83.

20. Hofauer B, Steffen A, Knopf A, et al. Adherence to upper-airway stimulation in the treatment of OSA. Chest 2018;153(2):574–5.

21. Hofauer B, Steffen A, Knopf A, et al. Patient experience with upper airway stimulation in the treatment of obstructive sleep apnea. Sleep Breath 2018. [Epub ahead of print].

22. Hasselbacher K, Hofauer B, Maurer JT, et al. Patient-reported outcome: results of the multicenter German post-market study. Eur Arch Otorhinolaryngol 2018;128(2):509–15.

23. Bowen AJ, Nowacki AS, Kominsky AH, et al. Voice and swallowing outcomes following hypoglossal nerve stimulation for obstructive sleep apnea. Am J Otolaryngol 2018;39(2):122–6.

24. Heiser C, Maurer JT, Steffen A. Functional outcome of tongue motions with selective hypoglossal nerve stimulation in patients with obstructive sleep apnea. Sleep Breath 2015;20(2):553–60.

25. Heiser C. Advanced titration to treat a floppy epiglottis in selective upper airway stimulation. Laryngoscope 2016;126(Suppl 7):S22–4.

26. Hofauer B, Strohl K, Knopf A, et al. Sonographic evaluation of tongue motions during upper airway stimulation for obstructive sleep apnea-a pilot study. Sleep Breath 2017;21(1):101–7.

27. Steffen A, Kilic A, König IR, et al. Tongue motion variability with changes of upper airway stimulation electrode configuration and effects on treatment outcomes. Laryngoscope 2018;128(8):1970–6.

28. Heiser C, Edenharter G, Bas M, et al. Palatoglossus coupling in selective upper airway stimulation. Laryngoscope 2017;127(10):E378–83.

29. Heiser C, Thaler E, Boon M, et al. Updates of operative techniques for upper airway stimulation. Laryngoscope 2016;126(Suppl 7):S12–6.

30. Heiser C, Thaler E, Soose RJ, et al. Technical tips during implantation of selective upper airway stimulation. Laryngoscope 2018;128(3):756–62.

31. Heiser C, Knopf A, Hofauer B. Surgical anatomy of the hypoglossal nerve: a new classification system for selective upper airway stimulation. Head Neck 2017;39(12):2371–80.

32. Heiser C, Hofauer B, Lozier L, et al. Nerve monitoring guided selective hypoglossal nerve stimulation in obstructive sleep apnea. Laryngoscope 2016;126(12):2852–8.

33. Kent DT, Lee JJ, Strollo PJ, et al. Upper airway stimulation for OSA: early adherence and outcome results of one center. Otolaryngol Head Neck Surg 2016;155(1):188–93.

34. Huntley C, Kaffenberger T, Doghramji K, et al. Upper airway stimulation for treatment of obstructive sleep apnea: an evaluation and comparison of outcomes at two academic centers. J Clin Sleep Med 2017;13(9):1075–9.

35. Boon M, Huntley C, Steffen A, et al. Upper airway stimulation for obstructive sleep apnea: results from the ADHERE registry. Otolaryngol Head Neck Surg 2018;159(2):379–85.

The Role of the Revised Stanford Protocol in Today's Precision Medicine

Stanley Yung-Chuan Liu, MD, DDS*,
Michael Awad, MD, FRCSC, Robert Riley, MD, DDS,
Robson Capasso, MD

KEYWORDS

- Riley-Powell protocol • Maxillomandibular advancement • Upper airway stimulation
- Stanford sleep surgery protocol • Obstructive sleep apnea

KEY POINTS

- From a tiered approach, the revised protocol functions on a continuum that is applicable to OSA as a chronic condition, and where procedures are elective.
- The revised protocol is defined by precision in patient selection, procedural selection, and procedural accuracy.
- Timing and indication for skeletal surgery is addressed with better understanding of sleep physiology and contemporary diagnostic modality including drug-induced sedation endoscopy.
- Maxillomandibular advancement and upper airway stimulation consistently demonstrate high rates of surgical success.

INTRODUCTION

Whereas the original Stanford protocol relied on a tiered approach to care to avoid unnecessary surgery, it did not address the issue of surgical relapse, a common concern among sleep medicine specialists. With 3 decades of experience since the original 2-tiered Powell-Riley protocol was introduced and the role of evolving skeletal techniques and upper airway stimulation (UAS), we are pleased to present our current protocol. This update includes an emphasis on facial skeletal development with an impact on function, including nasal breathing, as well as the incorporation of UAS. The increased versatility of palatopharyngoplasty as an adjunctive procedure for other procedures including UAS is also discussed.

JUSTIFICATION FOR SURGICAL MANAGEMENT OF OBSTRUCTIVE SLEEP APNEA

The health care burden of undiagnosed obstructive sleep apnea syndrome (OSAS) was approximately US$149.6 billion in 2015. The largest component of this burden is lost productivity accounting for US$86.9 billion or US$6366 per person. The remainder of this enormous financial burden is composed of medical and psychiatric comorbidities as well as motor vehicle and occupational accidents.

OSAS is associated with neurocognitive and pathophysiologic sequelae with surgical intervention aimed to reduce disease-associated morbidity. Patients who suffer from excessive daytime sleepiness as a result of OSAS exhibit

Disclosure Statement: No disclosures.
Division of Sleep Surgery, Department of Otolaryngology, Stanford University School of Medicine, 801 Welch Road, Stanford, California 94304, USA
* Corresponding author.
E-mail address: ycliu@stanford.edu

Sleep Med Clin 14 (2019) 99–107
https://doi.org/10.1016/j.jsmc.2018.10.013
1556-407X/19/© 2018 Elsevier Inc. All rights reserved.

emotional lability and impaired social functioning, and are predisposed to automobile accidents.[1,2] Finally, patients with OSAS suffer morbidity associated with hypertension, congestive heart failure, myocardial infarction, cardiac arrhythmias, and cerebrovascular disease. Surgical intervention is aimed at reducing upper airway collapsibility during sleep and mitigating hypoxemia, respiratory events, and normalizing sleep architecture.[3]

INDICATIONS FOR SURGERY

Although the original surgical indications remain a key component of management, shifting focus has turned toward the reduction of disease burden with the aim to manage OSAS as a chronic condition rather than aim for cure (**Box 1**). Specific to the new protocol, growing individuals such as teenagers and young adults are of particular interest to introduce interventions early that can help to improve facial skeletal growth and thus reduce the burden of disease in later adulthood.[4]

PATIENT SELECTION, PHYSICAL EXAMINATION, AND DIAGNOSTIC IMAGING

Achieving maximal surgical success depends on accurate patient phenotyping with targeted physical examination and diagnostic studies. Full head and neck examination, polysomnography data, fiberoptic nasopharyngoscopy, drug-induced sedation endoscopy (DISE), and diagnostic imaging are used to phenotype airway anatomy. Attention should be paid to identifying potential obstruction sites, including nasal airway, palate/velopharynx, lateral pharyngeal wall, the base of tongue, and the epiglottis.

Of growing importance are objective patient measures including Epworth sleepiness scores, NOSE Scores, and fatigue severity scales.

A level 1, or attended, overnight polysomnography remains the gold standard for diagnosis of obstructive sleep apnea. Increasingly, this modality is being replaced with a home sleep test. However, caution should be taken by the diagnostician because ambulatory studies may underestimate disease severity and surgical success can only be determined by comparing like with like diagnostic studies. Beyond the apnea-hypopnea index, the sleep surgeon should take special interest in the oxygen desaturation index and nadir to better characterize disease severity.[5] Care should be taken to pay attention to the various definitions of hypopnea that have evolved in recent years.[6] The oxygen desaturation index has been demonstrated to correlate more strongly with medical sequelae of OSAS than the apnea-hypopnea index alone, in particular cardiovascular morbidity.[7,8] In the current Stanford protocol, focus is also given to patient-reported outcomes, including satisfaction and subjective response to therapy.

Continuous positive airway pressure intolerance secondary to nasal obstruction is a key area of focus in the current Stanford protocol. Previously, we showed that 26% of patients who are intolerant of continuous positive airway pressure have nasal obstruction associated with posterior septal deviation that was only recognized by nasopharyngoscopy.[9] Therefore, examination with anterior rhinoscopy alone is not sufficient in this subset of affected individuals.[10]

When examining the oral cavity, including both the soft and hard palates, lateral pharyngeal walls, tongue base, and the hypopharynx, previously described grading systems by Mallampati and Freidman remain of clinical value. Characteristic skeletal morphologies have been identified in patients with OSAS. Of considerable interest, palatal width and height have been demonstrated to be reduced in both male and female patients with OSAS.[11,12]

Riley and Powell used the lateral cephalogram to correlate hyoid position, soft palate length, posterior airway space, and maxillofacial position, with studies showing cephalometry compares favorably with computed tomographic scans of the upper airway.[13] Static examination of the

---

Box 1
Surgical indications

- Apnea/hypopnea index of >20[a] events per hour of sleep
- Oxygen desaturation nadir, 90%
- Esophageal pressure more negative than −10 cm H_2O
- Cardiovascular derangements (arrhythmia, hypertension)
- Neurobehavioral symptoms (excessive daytime sleepiness)
- Failure of medical management
- Anatomic sites of obstruction (nose, palate, tongue base)

[a] Surgery may be indicated with an apnea/hypopnea index of less than 20 if accompanied by excessive daytime fatigue.

From Powell NB, Riley RW, Guilleminault C. Surgical management of sleep-disordered breathing. In: Kryger MH, Roth T, Dement WC, editors. Principles and practices of sleep medicine. 4th edition. Philadelphia: Elsevier Saunders; 2005. p. 1081–97; with permission.

airway using various modes of imaging is partially replaced by DISE. DISE is required for UAS candidacy. Patients who demonstrate a pattern of concentric collapse at the velum are not considered candidates for implantation. This topic is further discussed elsewhere in this article.

Our study of perioperative DISE findings after maxillomandibular advancement (MMA) has also identified likely responders to MMA-first intervention.[14] DISE has also allowed a greater understanding of the role of epiglottis collapse in the pathophysiology of OSAS.[15]

THE ORIGINAL PHASE I AND PHASE II STANFORD PROTOCOL

The original phase I and phase II Stanford Protocol was created as a means of targeting the multilevel obstruction typical of patients with OSAS while avoiding unnecessary surgical intervention (**Fig. 1**). The procedures comprising phase I and phase II of the protocol are described in **Box 2**. Classically, 6 months after undergoing the phase I protocol, patients would undergo repeat polysomnography and if surgical success (defined in **Box 3**) was achieved, no further intervention was required apart from routine follow-up. When phase I alone was not successful in achieving surgical success, the sleep surgeon could proceed to phase II of the protocol, encompassing MMA. For clarity, the terms maxillomandibular advancement osteotomy and MMA are interchangeable.

Approximately 60% of appropriately selected patients achieved surgical cure with phase I surgery alone, with overall response rates ranging from 42% to 75%.[16] Factors predisposing to surgical failure include a mean Respiratory Disturbance Index of greater than 60 events, Oxygen nadir greater than 70%, mandibular deficiency (sella nasion B point <75°) and morbid obesity (body mass index of >33 kg/m^2).

Patients who are incompletely treated by phase I surgery often have persistent hypopharyngeal obstruction. This level of obstruction classically involves complete collapse of the lateral pharyngeal walls. A proportion of these patients are subsequently able to tolerate positive airway pressure therapy after phase I surgery, an effect likely attributable to reduced nasal resistance. The remainder are offered MMA surgery, which has documented success rate of 90%.[16–18]

THE CURRENT STANFORD PROTOCOL

The current Stanford Protocol is outlined in **Fig. 2** and each component described herein.

Nasal Reconstruction

Nasal surgery aims to maintain nasal airway patency and minimize mouth breathing by treating septal deviation, turbinate hypertrophy, and/or nasal valve incompetence. Improving nasal breathing decreases associated mouth opening during sleep, which results in posterior

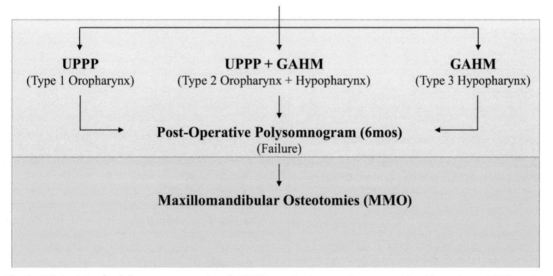

Presurgical Evaluation
(Physical Examination, Cephalometric Analysis, Fiberoptic Pharyngoscopy)

| UPPP | UPPP + GAHM | GAHM |
| (Type 1 Oropharynx) | (Type 2 Oropharynx + Hypopharynx) | (Type 3 Hypopharynx) |

Post-Operative Polysomnogram (6mos)
(Failure)

Maxillomandibular Osteotomies (MMO)

Fig. 1. Original stanford sleep surgery protocol. GAHM, genioglossus advancement hyoid myotomy; UPPP, uvulopalatopharyngoplasty. (*Adapted from* Riley RW, Powell NB, Guilleminault C. Obstructive sleep apnea syndrome: a surgical protocol for dynamic upper airway reconstruction. J Oral Maxillofac Surg 1993;51; with permission.)

Box 2
Powell–Riley protocol surgical procedures

Phase I

Nasal surgery (septoplasty, turbinate reduction, nasal valve grafting)

Tonsillectomy

Uvulopalatopharyngoplasty or uvulopalatal flap

Mandibular osteotomy with genioglossus advancement

Hyoid myotomy and suspension

Temperature-controlled radiofrequency[a]—inferior turbinates, palate, tongue base

Phase II

Maxillomandibular advancement osteotomy

Temperature-controlled radiofrequency[a]-tongue base

[a] Temperature-controlled radiofrequency is typically used as an adjunctive treatment. Select patients may choose temperature-controlled radiofrequency as primary treatment.
From Powell NB, Riley RW, Guilleminault C. Surgical management of sleep-disordered breathing. In: Kryger MH, Roth T, Dement WC, editors. Principles and practices of sleep medicine. 4th edition. Philadelphia: Elsevier Saunders; 2005. p. 1081–97; with permission.

displacement of the tongue into the hypopharyngeal airway and associated obstruction. Surgical options include septoplasty, turbinate reduction, or open septorhinoplasty with alar grafting. Although treating nasal obstruction does not cure

Box 3
Definition of surgical responders

- Apnea/hypopnea index of 20 events per hour of sleep[a]
- Oxygen desaturation nadir of greater than 90%
- Excessive daytime fatigue alleviated
- Normalization of sleep architecture
- Response equivalent to continuous positive airway pressure on full-night titration

[a] A reduction of the apnea/hypopnea index by 50% or more is considered a cure if the preoperative apnea/hypopnea index is less than 20.
From Powell NB, Riley RW, Guilleminault C. Surgical management of sleep-disordered breathing. In: Kryger MH, Roth T, Dement WC, editors. Principles and practices of sleep medicine. 4th edition. Philadelphia: Elsevier Saunders; 2005. p. 1081–97; with permission.

OSAS, it improves the quality of life and sleep significantly. Furthermore, it has been shown to improve adherence with continuous positive airway pressure.[19]

Distraction Osteogenesis Maxillary Expansion

An emerging concept in OSAS surgery, the concept of distraction osteogenesis maxillary expansion originated from the identification of a subset of patients with persistent subjective nasal obstruction, with a classical phenotype of high-arched and narrow maxilla, without associated turbinate hypertrophy, septal deviation, or nasal valve collapse. Evidence from the pediatric population demonstrates resolution of OSAS with the use of orthodontic expanders, particularly in children with persistent disease after adenotonsillectomy.[4,20,21] The proposed mechanism for improvement in sleep-disordered breathing from maxillary expansion is increased nasal floor width with associated decreased nasal resistance. By widening the maxillary transverse dimension, it has been hypothesized that the increased oral cavity space allows for a more superior and anterior position of the tongue and a greater posterior pharyngeal airway space, with a subsequent decrease in airway obstruction.[22]

The procedure involves the creation of Lefort I osteotomies bilaterally in conjunction with splitting the midpalatal suture and subsequent application of an orthognathic maxillary expander. Indications for distraction osteogenesis maxillary expansion are described in **Box 4**.

Palate Surgery: Tonsillectomy and Pharyngoplasty

The workhorse of sleep apnea surgery, the uvulopalatal flap, was performed alone or in conjunction with other procedures as part of phase I. The procedure enlarges the retropalatal airway via the excision of tonsil tissue (if present), trimming and reorienting the anterior and posterior tonsillar pillars, and excising a portion of the uvula and soft palate. Uvulopalatopharyngoplasty is an excellent technique to treat isolated retropalatal obstruction. However, there is often a stigma associated with this procedure owing to its intense postoperative pain and variable success rates. Sher and colleagues[23] documented that uvulopalatopharyngoplasty had a cure rate of 39%. Unrecognized hypopharyngeal obstruction was believed to be the primary reason for this high failure rate.

A reversible uvulopalatal flap as described by Riley and Powell remains a viable option with good short- and long-term outcomes and minimal complication rates.[24] Clinical experience has

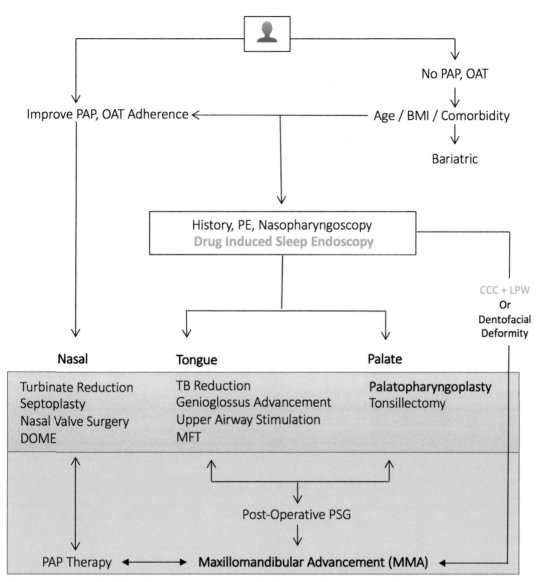

Fig. 2. Current Stanford sleep surgery protocol. BMI, body mass index; CCC, complete concentric collapse; DOME, distraction osteogenesis maxillary expansion; LPW, lateral pharyngeal wall; MFT, myofunctional therapy; OAT, oral appliance therapy; PAP, positive airway pressure; PE, physical examination; PSG, polysomnography; TB, tongue base.

demonstrated palate techniques requiring minimal muscular relocation and maximum tissue preservation to reduce morbidity while improving patient satisfaction. Notably, the 15-year follow-up has shown significant and sustained decreases in oxygen desaturation index values and patient reported improvement in daytime sleepiness.[25]

Of interest in the updated Stanford Protocol is the role of palatopharyngoplasty in converting patients with complete concentric collapse at the velum on DISE. After undergoing palatopharyngoplasty, the majority of patients have been shown to convert to an anterior-posterior pattern

of collapse. This anterior-posterior pattern of collapse is an indication for UAS implantation.

Upper Airway Stimulation

Of emerging interest, UAS has gained traction in the United States since approval in 2014. The concept of UAS focuses on the genioglossus muscle as a key protrusor of the tongue musculature. A number of animal studies between 1989 and 1996 identified a link between stimulation of the hypoglossal nerve and upper airway dilatation, airway resistance, and airway stability.[26–29] After

---

Box 4
Indications for distraction osteogenesis maxillary expansion surgery

- Patients with obstructive sleep apnea syndrome who present with absolute skeletal transverse hypoplasia and an associated cross-bite
- Mild obstructive sleep apnea syndrome or upper airway resistance syndrome with complaints of persistent nasal obstruction and associated narrow, high-arched palate who have (1) undergone previous nasal surgery or (2) do not present with significant septal deviation, inferior turbinate hypertrophy, or nasal valve collapse

---

early unsuccessful attempts at electrical stimulation, the Inspire I and II trials demonstrated promising results during an early development race between Apnex (St. Paul, MN), ImThera Medical (San Diego, CA), and Inspire (Maple Grove, MN). These experiences culminated in the large multicenter phase II/III trial known as the STAR trial, which was completed in 2014. One hundred twenty-six patients were enrolled with the criteria for inclusion listed in **Box 5**. The INSPIRE system consists of 3 parts: a stimulation electrode in the form of a cuff that envelopes the anterior (protrusor) branches of the hypoglossal nerve, a pleural pressure sensing lead, and an implantable pulse generator. The implantable electrodes allows a range of freedom in postoperative titration to optimize control of breathing events.[30] Indications for UAS, adapted and updated since the STAR trial, are described in **Box 5**.

The mid- to long-term data on UAS is promising. Five-year follow-up has demonstrated sustained benefit in obstructive sleep apnea severity and patient-reported outcome measures.[31]

Box 5
Indications for upper airway stimulation

- Moderate to severe obstructive sleep apnea syndrome (apnea-hypopnea index of 15–65)
- Less than 25% central apneas
- Body mass index of less than 32
- No evidence of concentric collapse of the velum on drug-induced sedation endoscopy

Adapted from Woodson BT, Soose RJ, Gillespie MB, et al. Three-year outcomes of cranial nerve stimulation for obstructive sleep apnea: the STAR trial. Otolaryngol Head Neck Surg 2016;154; with permission.

Tongue Base Surgery

The human tongue is divided into (1) the blade or tip (anterior to the frenulum), (2) the body (which extends from the frenulum to the circumvallate papillae), and (3) the base of the tongue, which is posterior to the circumvallate papillae. This complex organ, which functions as a muscular hydrostat, has become of great interest to the modern sleep surgeon. Tongue base obstruction has been demonstrated to play a role in OSAS in one-third of moderate to severe cases. As a result, a multitude of surgical options for managing the tongue base have been described These techniques include cold and hot resection, laser reduction, radiofrequency ablation, and coblation. Most prevalent of these is transoral robotic surgery. The first transoral robotic surgery case for OSAS was performed by Vicini and Montevcchi in Forli, Italy in 2008. A growing body of evidence, recently bolstered by Garas and colleagues,[32] has reported transoral robotic surgery efficacy rates of greater than 75% in the nonobese patients with OSAS, and 50% of nonmorbidly obese patients with OSAS.[33]

Genioglossus Advancement

Genioglossus advancement is typically performed as part of the phase I surgery to stabilize the tongue base and limit posterior displacement of the tongue into the hypopharyngeal airway during sleep.[29,34] The genial tubercle, genioglossus muscle, and tongue base are advanced anteriorly by creating a rectangular osteotomy of the anterior mandible, which is then advanced and secured to the inferior portion of the mandible. Many variations of Riley and Powell's original technique have been described.[35–38] In select patients, genioglossus advancement incorporating the inferior border of the mandible is appropriate for both tongue base stability via suprahyoid muscle tension and facial aesthetics. This procedure is considered a conservative technique that does not change occlusion or jaw position and can be designed to improve facial aesthetics where desired. Recent data demonstrate dwindling interest in isolated genioglossus advancement in the sleep surgery literature.[39] More recently, virtual surgical planning has been used to personalize the osteotomy for the individual patient while mitigating known risks of the procedure.[40] These measures include avoiding damage to the dental roots, mental nerve injury, and mandibular fractures.[41] Acknowledging previous challenges with the procedure, we developed a simple method of preoperative surgical planning with osteotomy guides that allow accurate osteotomies and planned fixation.

Maxillomandibular Advancement

A number of updates to the role and technique of MMA in the Stanford protocol have been accomplished. This includes improved understanding of the importance of counterclockwise rotation of the maxilla during advancement in improving functional outcomes. This allows for a greater degree of advancement while maintaining and improving facial aesthetics. Nasal function and the subsequent need for revision procedures is reducing by paying particular attention to performing primary septoplasty and expansion of the piriform rim during Le Fort I osteotomy at the time of MMA surgery.[42]

Our updated MMA protocol has allowed for a significant decrease in postoperative pain and faster return to function with patients typically on a purée diet by the third week postoperatively. Patients are not in maxillomandibular fixation postoperatively and are placed in less intrusive guiding elastics. Surgery-first or surgery-early technique with regard to orthodontic treatment allows for excellent airway outcomes with large-scale advancements, which have been shown to be correlated with surgical success.[17]

Update: Phase II Preceding Phase I Surgery

Two categories of patients can benefit from proceeding to Phase II (MMA) without first undergoing phase I surgery.

1. Patients with OSAS and concurrent dentofacial deformity

Patients who have a coexisting indication for orthognathic/corrective jaw surgery are indicated for proceeding directly to MMA surgery to concurrently improve speech and mastication function.

2. Patients with moderate to severe OSAS without dentofacial deformity with
   a. Complete lateral pharyngeal wall collapse on DISE,
   b. Low hyoid position and obtuse cervicomental angle, and
   c. High inclination of the occlusal plane.

Previous static and dynamic airway study demonstrates MMA results in significantly improved airway stability at the level of the lateral pharyngeal walls, an anatomic site that is difficult to address with soft tissue surgery alone.[43] For patients who demonstrate severe/complete lateral pharyngeal wall collapse on DISE, MMA is offered upfront. The patient should be counseled that phase I surgery or other medical interventions may still be required to fully manage OSAS.

SUMMARY

Although the original Stanford Protocol remains the cornerstone of surgical decision making in patients with OSAS, a number of key surgical innovations have been developed further adding to the arsenal of the modern sleep surgeon. These include special considerations such as treatment relapse, upfront MMA (phase II surgery), and modern techniques such as UAS and distraction osteogenesis maxillary expansion.

The evolving Stanford Protocol continues to play a central role in collaboration with medical therapies in the management of OSAS. A concerted effort between Sleep Medicine specialists and sleep surgeons informs a patient-centered future for our specialty where we are able to provide a range of therapeutic options to best suit the patient's goals for treatment.

ACKNOWLEDGMENTS

The authors would like to acknowledge the contributions of Howard Awad, MD, ABSM, for his contributions in reviewing and providing input on multiple iterations of this article. The authors would also like to acknowledge Nelson Powell, MD, DDS, for his contribution to development of the original Powell-Riley Protocol.

REFERENCES

1. Bonnet MH. Effect of sleep disruption on sleep, performance, and mood. Sleep 1985;8(1):11–9.
2. Powell NB, Schechtman KB, Riley RW, et al. Sleepy driving: accidents and injury. Otolaryngol Head Neck Surg 2016;126(3):217–27.
3. Liu SYC, Huon LK, Ruoff C, et al. Restoration of sleep architecture after maxillomandibular advancement: success beyond the apnea-hypopnea index. Int J Oral Maxillofac Surg 2017;46(12):1533–8.
4. Liu SY-C, Guilleminault C, Huon L-K, et al. Distraction osteogenesis maxillary expansion (DOME) for adult obstructive sleep apnea patients with high arched palate. Otolaryngol Head Neck Surg 2017; 157(2):345–8.
5. Lan M-C, Liu SYC, Lan M-Y, et al. Lateral pharyngeal wall collapse associated with hypoxemia in obstructive sleep apnea. Laryngoscope 2015;125(10): 2408–12.
6. Heinzer R, Vat S, Marques-Vidal P, et al. Prevalence of sleep-disordered breathing in the general population: the HypnoLaus study. Lancet Respir Med 2015; 3(4):310–8.
7. Punjabi NM, Newman AB, Young TB, et al. Sleep-disordered breathing and cardiovascular disease: an outcome-based definition of hypopneas. Am J Respir Crit Care Med 2008;177(10):1150–5.

8. Kendzerska T, Gershon AS, Hawker G, et al. Obstructive sleep apnea and risk of cardiovascular events and all-cause mortality: a decade-long historical cohort study. In: Patel A, editor. PLoS Med 2014; 11(2):e1001599.

9. Torre C, Capasso R, Zaghi S, et al. High incidence of posterior nasal cavity obstruction in obstructive sleep apnea patients. Sleep Sci Pract 2017;1(1):286.

10. Camacho M, Zaghi S, Certal V, et al. Inferior turbinate classification system, grades 1 to 4: development and validation study. Laryngoscope 2015; 125(2):296–302.

11. Johal A, Conaghan C. Maxillary morphology in obstructive sleep apnea: a cephalometric and model study. Angle Orthod 2004;74(5):648–56.

12. Torre C, Zaghi S, Camacho M, et al. Hypopharyngeal evaluation in obstructive sleep apnea with awake flexible laryngoscopy: validation and updates to Cormack-Lehane and Modified Cormack-Lehane scoring systems. Clin Otolaryngol 2018;43(3):823–7.

13. Riley R, Powell N, Guilleminault C. Cephalometric roentgenograms and computerized tomographic scans in obstructive sleep apnea. Sleep 1986;9(4):514–5.

14. Liu SY-C, Huon L-K, Iwasaki T, et al. Efficacy of maxillomandibular advancement examined with drug-induced sleep endoscopy and computational fluid dynamics airflow modeling. Otolaryngol Head Neck Surg 2016;154(1):189–95.

15. Torre C, Camacho M, Liu SY-C, et al. Epiglottis collapse in adult obstructive sleep apnea: a systematic review. Laryngoscope 2016;126(2):515–23.

16. Riley RW, Powell NB, Guilleminault C. Obstructive sleep apnea syndrome: a review of 306 consecutively treated surgical patients. Otolaryngol Head Neck Surg 1993;108(2):117–25.

17. Holty J-EC, Guilleminault C. Maxillomandibular advancement for the treatment of obstructive sleep apnea: a systematic review and meta-analysis. Sleep Med Rev 2010;14(5):287–97.

18. Zaghi S, Holty J-EC, Certal V, et al. Maxillomandibular advancement for treatment of obstructive sleep apnea. JAMA Otolaryngol Head Neck Surg 2016; 142(1):58–9.

19. Camacho M, Riaz M, Capasso R, et al. The effect of nasal surgery on continuous positive airway pressure device use and therapeutic treatment pressures: a systematic review and meta-analysis. Sleep 2015;38(2):279–86.

20. Pirelli P, Saponara M, Guilleminault C. Rapid maxillary expansion in children with obstructive sleep apnea syndrome. Sleep 2004;27(4):761–6.

21. Cistulli PA, Palmisano RG, Poole MD. Treatment of obstructive sleep apnea syndrome by rapid maxillary expansion. Sleep 1998;21(8):831–5.

22. Vinha PP, Eckeli AL, Faria AC, et al. Effects of surgically assisted rapid maxillary expansion on obstructive sleep apnea and daytime sleepiness. Sleep Breath 2016;20(2):501–8.

23. Sher AE, Schechtman KB, Piccirillo JF. The efficacy of surgical modifications of the upper airway in adults with obstructive sleep apnea syndrome. Sleep 1996;19(2):156–77.

24. Neruntarat C. Uvulopalatal flap for obstructive sleep apnea: short-term and long-term results. Laryngoscope 2011;121(3):683–7.

25. Browaldh N, Friberg D, Svanborg E, et al. 15-year efficacy of uvulopalatopharyngoplasty based on objective and subjective data. Acta Otolaryngol 2011;131(12):1303–10.

26. Oliven A, Odeh M, Schnall RP. Improved upper airway patency elicited by electrical stimulation of the hypoglossus nerves. Respiration 1996;63(4): 213–6.

27. Yoo PB, Durand DM. Effects of selective hypoglossal nerve stimulation on canine upper airway mechanics. J Appl Physiol (1985) 2005;99(3):937–43.

28. Miki H, Hida W, Shindoh C, et al. Effects of electrical stimulation of the genioglossus on upper airway resistance in anesthetized dogs. Am Rev Respir Dis 1989;140(5):1279–84.

29. Song SA, Chang ET, Certal V, et al. Genial tubercle advancement and genioplasty for obstructive sleep apnea: a systematic review and meta-analysis. Laryngoscope 2017;127(4):984–92.

30. Woodson BT, Soose RJ, Gillespie MB, et al. Three-year outcomes of cranial nerve stimulation for obstructive sleep apnea: the STAR trial. Otolaryngol Head Neck Surg 2016;154(1):181–8.

31. Strollo PJ, Soose R, Badr M, et al. 0563 Upper airway stimulation for obstructive sleep apnea: objective and patient reported outcomes after five years of follow-up. Sleep 2017;40(suppl_1):A209.

32. Garas G, Kythreotou A, Georgalas C, et al. Is transoral robotic surgery a safe and effective multilevel treatment for obstructive sleep apnoea in obese patients following failure of conventional treatment(s)? Ann Med Surg (Lond) 2017;19:55–61.

33. Camacho M, Certal V, Capasso R. Comprehensive review of surgeries for obstructive sleep apnea syndrome. Braz J Otorhinolaryngol 2013;79(6):780–8.

34. Riley RW, Powell NB, Guilleminault C. Inferior sagittal osteotomy of the mandible with hyoid myotomy-suspension: a new procedure for obstructive sleep apnea. Otolaryngol Head Neck Surg 1986;94(5):589–93.

35. Riley R, Guilleminault C, Powell N, et al. Mandibular osteotomy and hyoid bone advancement for obstructive sleep apnea: a case report. Sleep 1984;7(1):79–82.

36. García Vega JR, de la Plata MM, Galindo N, et al. Genioglossus muscle advancement: a modification of the conventional technique. J Craniomaxillofac Surg 2014;42(3):239–44.

37. Lee NR, Madani M. Genioglossus muscle advancement techniques for obstructive sleep apnea. Atlas Oral Maxillofac Surg Clin North Am 2007;15(2): 179–92.

38. Hendler B, Silverstein K, Giannakopoulos H, et al. Mortised genioplasty in the treatment of obstructive sleep apnea: an historical perspective and modification of design. Sleep Breath 2001;5(4): 173–80.

39. Ishman SL, Ishii LE, Gourin CG. Temporal trends in sleep apnea surgery: 1993-2010. Laryngoscope 2014;124(5):1251–8.

40. Liu SY-C, Huon L-K, Zaghi S, et al. An accurate method of designing and performing individual-specific genioglossus advancement. Otolaryngol Head Neck Surg 2017;156(1):194–7.

41. Handler E, Hamans E, Goldberg AN, et al. Tongue suspension: an evidence-based review and comparison to hypopharyngeal surgery for OSA. Laryngoscope 2014;124(1):329–36.

42. Liu SY-C, Lee P-J, Awad M, et al. Corrective nasal surgery after maxillomandibular advancement for obstructive sleep apnea: experience from 379 cases. Otolaryngol Head Neck Surg 2017;157(1):156–9.

43. Soares D, Sinawe H, Folbe AJ, et al. Lateral oropharyngeal wall and supraglottic airway collapse associated with failure in sleep apnea surgery. Laryngoscope 2012;122(2):473–9.

Oral Appliances in the Management of Obstructive Sleep Apnea

Jing Hao Ng, BDS (Singapore), MDS Orthodontics (Singapore), MOrth RCS (Edinburgh, UK)*, Mimi Yow, BDS (Singapore), FDS RCS (Edinburgh), MSc (London) (Orthodontics), FAMS (Craniofacial Orthodontics)

KEYWORDS

- OSA • Oral appliance • Mandibular advancement • Tongue stabilizer

KEY POINTS

- The concept in oral appliances for obstructive sleep apnea (OSA) management is protrusion of the mandible and/or tongue for structural effects on the upper airway.
- The upper airway is a muscular tube and its dimensions are enlarged with mandibular and tongue advancement.
- Protrusion of the mandible and tongue stretches the muscles, thereby reducing upper airway collapsibility with airway shape change and increase in muscle tone.
- Oral appliances are effective and evidence-based options in managing OSA.

TYPES OF ORAL APPLIANCES

The primary oral appliance (OA) used in obstructive sleep apnea (OSA) treatment is the mandibular advancement device (MAD). MADs may be either an over-the-counter stock device or customized for individual patients. MADs come in various designs and materials, but most comprise upper and lower splints mounted over the dentition as either a 1-piece monoblock (**Fig. 1**) or a 2-piece biblock (**Fig. 2**). Connectors or blocks relate the upper and lower splints in a biblock to protrude the mandible in a forward position during sleep.[1]

Tongue-retaining devices, or tongue-stabilizing devices (TSDs) (**Fig. 3**), are a second type of OA, which displace the tongue anteriorly and may be customized or come in different stock sizes. TSDs use negative pressure and salivary adhesion to hold onto the tongue and anterior lip shields to elongate and reposition the tongue in a more forward position independent of the mandible during sleep, thereby opening the oropharyngeal airway.[1,2]

TSDs have similar efficacy as MADs but poorer compliance. More than 90% of patients preferred MADs over TSDs for OA therapy.[3] The evidence base is stronger for MADs and considerably lower for TSDs.[2,4,5]

ORAL APPLIANCE EFFECTS ON AIRWAY
Cross-Sectional Area

Airway imaging with cone-beam computed tomography, magnetic resonance imaging and nasal endoscopy showed anteroposterior (AP) mandibular protrusion predominantly increases the caliber of the airway at the retropalatal area via lateral expansion and displacement of parapharyngeal fat pads[2,6–13] while the tongue and tongue-base muscles shift forward.[2,9,13]

The lateral widening from AP movement is attributed to stretching of soft tissue connections

Disclosure Statement: The authors declare no conflicts of interest and no funding was received in the preparation of this article.

Department of Orthodontics, National Dental Centre Singapore, 5 Second Hospital Avenue, Singapore 168938, Singapore

* Corresponding author.

E-mail address: ng.jing.hao@singhealth.com.sg

Sleep Med Clin 14 (2019) 109–118
https://doi.org/10.1016/j.jsmc.2018.10.012

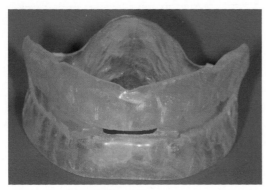

Fig. 1. Monoblock of 1-piece MAD. (*Courtesy of* the Orthodontic Laboratory in the National Dental Centre of Singapore, Singapore.)

between the tongue, soft palate, and lateral pharyngeal walls.[11,14,15] Dynamic MRI suggests a direct connection between lateral pharyngeal walls and the ramus, postulated to be the pterygomandibular raphe.[13]

TSDs increase airway AP diameter to a greater degree than MADs, and traction on intrapharyngeal connections through the tongue base additionally increases the lateral dimension of the airway. Compared with MADs, TSDs produce greater increases in retropalatal and retroglossal cross-sectional area (CSA). This is attributed to greater anterior tongue movement with TSDs.[2]

Other Effects

Lateral expansion with both MADs and TSDs promotes an elliptical cross-sectional shape with a

transverse long axis.[2] A small but significant decrease in upper airway length has been found with MAD use,[2] which may counteract the airway length increase from lying supine demonstrated in OSA patients.[16]

Electromyography shows that MADs increase activation of masseter, lateral pterygoid, genioglossus, and geniohyoid muscles. It is postulated that on top of the purely structural anatomic effects of MADs, increased neuromuscular activation contributes to upper airway patency.[17–19]

Collapsibility

Morphologic increase in CSA, change in cross-sectional shape, decrease in airway length, and neuromuscular activation with MAD may contribute to reduced collapsibility.[2,12,20] Empirically, a significant reduction in upper airway collapsibility in stage 2 and stage 3 sleep was observed with MAD use. Improvement in collapsibility was significantly greater in complete responders than in partial responders or nonresponders.[21] Airway collapsibility may have a dose-dependent relationship with mandibular advancement.[10]

ORAL APPLIANCE EFFECTS ON OBSTRUCTIVE SLEEP APNEA COMPARED WITH CONTINUOUS POSITIVE AIRWAY PRESSURE

Continuous positive airway pressure (CPAP) and MADs are chronic, noninvasive, symptomatic treatments for OSA that do not treat the underlying

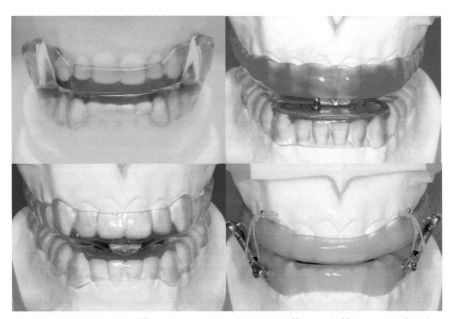

Fig. 2. Biblock or 2-piece MADs with different connectors. (*Courtesy of* [*upper left*] SomnoMed, Sydney, Australia; and [*upper right*, *lower left*, and *lower right*] Orthodontic Master, Singapore.)

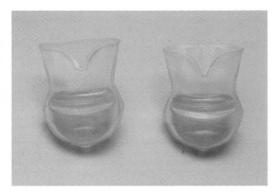

Fig. 3. TSD. (*Courtesy of* Innovative Health Technologies Ltd, Dunedin, New Zealand.)

anatomic basis of the condition. Pneumatic splinting of the airway with CPAP is acknowledged as the gold standard for treatment of OSA, although MAD has been progressively recommended with each iteration of the American Academy of Sleep Medicine (AASM) guidelines.[4,22,23] The latest AASM guidelines do not specify a particular disease severity for MAD use due to lack of evidence relating MAD efficacy to disease severity.[4]

Apnea-Hypopnea Index

MADs are efficacious in reducing apnea-hypopnea index (AHI) although there is individual variability.[24] A nonlinear dose-dependent relationship with degree of advancement is reported.[25–30]

The efficacy of CPAP over MAD in reducing AHI is well established and has been consistently reported by meta-analyses comparing the 2,[4,31–34] even with increasing numbers of primary studies. According to the AASM/American Academy of Dental Sleep Medicine (AADSM) task force, CPAP is significantly better than MAD at reducing AHI scores (difference of 6.24 events per hour).[4] A recent meta-analysis of 14 randomized controlled trials reported that CPAP reduced AHI by an additional 8.43 events per hour over MAD.[34]

Oxygenation

MADs are efficacious in improving minimum arterial oxygen saturation (Sao_2), and the improvement has been reported to have a nonlinear dose-dependent relationship with degree of advancement.[10]

Similar to AHI, the finding of better improvement in Sao_2 with CPAP over MAD has been consistently reported.[4,31,32,34] The AASM/AADSM task force reported that CPAP is slightly better at improving oxygenation (Sao_2 difference of 3.11%) compared with MADs.[4] More recently, a significant effect on Sao_2 in favor of CPAP was reported.[34]

Compliance

Comparing subjective self-reported MAD compliance with objective recorded CPAP compliance, MAD compliance is better. The AASM/AADSM task force reported that MADs were used 0.70 more hours per night than CPAP.[4] Objective measurements of OA usage after 3 months of OA treatment ranged from a mean of 6.4 hours to 6.6 hours per night.[35,36] A meta-analysis of 6 studies encompassing both subjective and objective MAD compliance measures reported an additional 1.1 hours per night use of MAD over CPAP.[33]

A majority of crossover trials report that MADs are preferred to CPAP, which may imply better patient compliance with MADs.[4,37,38] Depending on OSA severity and total sleep time, less than ideal compliance with CPAP can substantially decrease its effectiveness. Better MAD compliance over CPAP could be why health outcomes of the 2 treatment modalities are similar despite better CPAP efficacy at reducing AHI and increasing oxygenation.[37]

Subjective Sleepiness

MADs improve subjective daytime sleepiness measured by Epworth Sleepiness Scale (ESS) scores significantly.[39]

Despite better efficacy with CPAP than MADs in reducing AHI and improving Sao_2, differences in ESS scores are more ambiguous. A network meta-analysis of 67 studies found that CPAP and MADs are both effective in reducing excessive daytime sleepiness as assessed by the ESS, but CPAP is likely to be more effective than MADs, with a greater reduction in ESS by an average of 0.8 points.[40] Other reviews have reported either similar outcomes[4,32] or slightly better outcomes with CPAP.[33,34]

Function and Quality of Life

Aside from long-term health effects, untreated OSA also affects health-related quality of life, with hypersomnolence impacting ability to function.[41] Function and quality of life are commonly measured using both the sleep-specific Functional Outcomes of Sleep Questionnaire (FOSQ) and generic Medical Outcomes Study 36-Item Short Form Health Survey (SF-36). MADs are associated with improvements in FOSQ subscale and total scores as well as SF-36 scores.[4,42,43]

Minimal difference was found between CPAP and MAD with respect to improvements in daytime functional outcomes measured by SF-36 and FOSQ scores.[4] This finding was corroborated in a meta-analysis,[44] with direct comparisons as well as network meta-analysis showing no significant difference in treatment outcomes between CPAP and MAD in the mental and physical components of SF-36. Other meta-analyses have also reported no difference in FOSQ or SF-36 scores.[31–34]

Cardiovascular Effects

Meta-analyses by multiple groups have found MADs to be the equivalent of CPAP at reducing blood pressure in adults with OSA.[4,34,45–47] A network meta-analysis reported that CPAP was associated with a reduction in systolic blood pressure of 2.5 mm Hg and diastolic blood pressure reduction of 2.0 mm Hg. MADs were associated with reduction in systolic blood pressure of 2.1 mm Hg and diastolic blood pressure of 1.9 mm Hg. There was no significant difference between CPAP and MADs.[40]

Studies on other cardiovascular markers (heart rate variability, circulating cardiovascular biomarkers, endothelial function, and arterial stiffness) were deemed heterogeneous and inconclusive.[46]

Mortality

A prospective cohort study on long-term cardiovascular mortality in 208 subjects found CPAP and MAD equally effective in reducing the risk of fatal cardiovascular events in patients with severe OSA, despite higher residual AHI for MAD compared with CPAP users (16.3 vs 4.5 events per hour). There was no difference in the cumulative cardiovascular mortality between OSA patients treated with CPAP or MAD and that of the nonapneic controls, suggesting effective symptomatic treatment with either modality despite differences in residual AHI.[48] This outcome, however, is from a single observational study. More longitudinal studies with better methodology are needed to answer key questions on cardiovascular morbidity and mortality outcomes.[46,48]

ORAL APPLIANCE ADVERSE EFFECTS

Similar to efficacy, adverse side effects have a dose-dependent relationship with protrusion.[29] A balance must be struck between efficacy and side effects because more adverse effects reduce long-term compliance,[35,49] resulting in patients terminating MAD therapy.[50,51] Most adverse effects caused by MADs are mild and transient, occur during the initial phase of therapy, and tend to resolve with time.[51,52]

Dental Effects

Long-term use of OAs leads to occlusal changes. A meta-analysis reported a significant increase in lower incisor inclination by 2.07°, resulting in 0.99-mm decrease in overjet (OJ) and 1.0-mm decrease in overbite (OB). A greater decrease in OJ and OB was associated with longer treatment. There was no significant change in the upper incisor inclination or interincisal angle.[53]

Due to the lower incisor inclination change and attendant decrease in OJ and OB, there was significant increase in anterior crossbites,[54] increase in mandibular arch width, and reduction in lower arch crowding.[54,55] Maxillary arch width increase and upper arch decrowding also have been reported.[55] A decrease in posterior occlusal contacts[54,56–58] may result in a transient difficulty with chewing.[51] Although the magnitude of dental changes are small, they may be significant to patient perception of developing dental malocclusion.[59]

Craniofacial Changes

A meta-analysis of skeletal changes from MAD use reported no significant skeletal changes.[53] Other investigators, however, report significant increase in lower and total anterior facial height from long-term MAD use of more than 2 years.[60,61]

Temporomandibular Joint Disorders

Transient muscle soreness and temporomandibular joint (TMJ) discomfort have been reported after MAD use, especially during the initial titration period.[3,51] A 5-year follow-up study of MAD patients found mild, temporary subjective side effects, such as muscular or TMJ discomfort, but no changes in temporomandibular disorder prevalence using the Research Diagnostic Criteria for Temporomandibular Disorders.[57]

Other Effects

Other MAD side effects include increased salivation, more frequent and excessive dry mouth, tongue discomfort, and a sense of suffocation.[3,35,51] TSD side effects include excess salivation, drooling, dry mouth, and soft tissue irritation.[3]

PREDICTING AND IMPROVING ORAL APPLIANCE TREATMENT RESPONSE

Although most patients show an increased airway CSA with mandibular advancement, a minority of patients show no change or even a decreased CSA.[9,12] MAD is a primarily structural treatment[9] for a heterogeneous condition with nonanatomic etiology in up to 56% of patients.[62,63] Consequently, MAD treatment completely resolves AHI to fewer than 5 events per hour in only 36% to 70% of OSA patients.[24,38] Patients of female gender, younger age, smaller neck circumference, lower body mass index, lower AHI, and supine-dependent OSA are predicted to have better treatment success with MADs.[38,50,64,65] For TSDs, the best predictor of success is believed to be the presence of a single-site airway obstruction in supine-dependent OSA.[1]

There is currently no validated clinical method to reliably differentiate responders from nonresponders.[24] Uncertainty of MAD treatment response is exacerbated by cost of treatment.[66] The literature lacks consensus in successful treatment outcome, with a majority of success criteria used in research not meshing with clinical definitions of OSA severity. Discordant success criteria makes comparing results of different studies difficult.[67] Prospective trials are under way to determine predictive potential of wakeful nasoendoscopy with Müller maneuver, drug-induced sleep endoscopy (DISE), and computational fluid dynamics.[68,69] In the meantime, careful diagnosis and patient selection can increase the chances of success.

Cephalometry

Classically, shorter soft palate length, larger retropalatal airway space, lower hyoid bone position, and a smaller mandible are associated with favorable MAD treatment response.[1,65] Two recent systematic reviews,[70,71] however, exploring cephalometric predictors for MAD response found a majority of observational studies on cephalometric predictors had flawed designs and failed to control for known confounding factors such as age, gender, body mass index, and baseline AHI. Definitions of treatment success were inconsistent, and heterogeneity in design prevented data synthesis and meta-analysis. Cephalometric parameters warranting further study included mandibular plane angle, hyoid to mandibular plane distance, and soft palate length.

Mandibular Advancement Device Design

Customized versus noncustomized
Both customized and noncustomized MADs reduce AHI in adult patients with OSA, but meta-analysis by the AASM/AADSM task force shows the improvements to be far greater in customized than noncustomized, with an AHI reduction of 13.89 events compared with 6.28 events per hour.[4] Noncustomized MADs do not improve minimum Sao_2, whereas customized MADs increase Sao_2 by 3.22%.[4] They also do not reduce ESS scores to any significant level,[72] whereas modest improvements in ESS scores can be expected from customized MADs.[4]

Titratable versus nontitratable
Both custom titratable and custom nontitratable MADs reduce AHI, improve Sao_2 and reduce ESS scores, with meta-analyses by the AASM/AADSM task force showing the improvements to be approximately equivalent. Titratable MADs are recommended, however, over nontitratable MADs because the confidence interval for the effect of custom, titratable MADs is considerably smaller than for custom, nontitratable MADs.[4]

Due to dose-dependent effects, a clinical titration can improve MAD response and increase the amount of achievable protrusion. This is only possible with titratable MADs.[27]

Therapeutic Diagnosis

Visualizing airway response
Treatment response to MAD can be estimated by visualizing airway response to mandibular protrusion or tongue thrust with nasoendoscopy or MRI in awake supine patients, or in patients using DISE. An increase in velopharyngeal CSA with mandibular advancement was significantly associated with greater AHI reduction with MADs.[8,9,73,74] This was not fully predictive, however, with some patients without velopharyngeal widening showing high AHI reductions and vice versa.[2,73]

Müller maneuver during nasoendoscopy induced significantly greater collapse in velopharyngeal and oropharyngeal CSA in MAD nonresponders than responders. With mandibular advancement, Müller maneuver induced a significantly greater collapse at all airway levels in nonresponders.[8]

On MRI, TSD responders showed a greater increase with TSD in AP diameter, minimum and mean CSA, and volume compared with nonresponders.[2]

Mandibular advancement device titration using polysomnography
Due to the dose-dependent relationship between efficacy and protrusion, increasing protrusion can increase treatment response in OSA patients. Conventional titration protocols use subjective symptoms to adjust mandibular advancement over several months and an outcome polysomnography (PSG) to confirm efficacy. There is no consensus, however, on an optimal titration protocol.[67]

Manually increasing MAD advancement during overnight PSG can increase therapeutic efficacy of mandibular protrusion while reducing the number of titration visits required by most therapeutic protocols. After a clinical titration period, overnight MAD titration with PSG using the final MAD increased treatment response by an additional 9.9% to 30.4% of study subjects.[28,75] Disappointing outcomes were reported, however, using an interim MAD without a period of clinical titration because efficacy of the interim MAD was not translated to the final MAD.[76]

Overnight MAD titration with PSG may require large single-night mandibular advancements to relieve respiratory events, in contrast to slow titration with conventional protocols. Significant jaw discomfort was noted with PSG titration without prior MAD use[76] but was not reported by patients who had an adaptation period with conventional clinical MAD titration.[28]

Remote-controlled mandibular positioners

Using remote-controlled mandibular positioners (RCMPs) for single-night titration of MADs is similar to overnight MAD titration with PSG, with the advantage of adjustment done remotely without waking the patient or removing the appliance. Sleep architecture is maintained while protruding the mandible progressively until respiratory events are eliminated.[26,77–80]

RCMPs can determine an effective target protrusion that is correlated with successful MAD treatment, may be able to identify nonresponders early, and reduce the number of titration reviews needed compared with conventional titration protocols.[81] RCMP titration, however, necessitates large single-night mandibular advancements, which can cause significant jaw discomfort.[26]

Combination Therapy

Mandibular advancement device and tongue-stabilizing devices

Because TSDs have somewhat different anatomic effects on the airway compared with MADs,[2] combining the therapies using a novel hybrid appliance resulted in augmentative treatment effects. Tongue suction with 6 mm mandibular protrusion produced better treatment response than 8 mm mandibular protrusion alone.[30] Combination therapy might improve OA treatment response and prove useful in patients with limited mandibular protrusion.

Mandibular advancement device and continuous positive airway pressure

Combining MAD and CPAP lowered the therapeutic CPAP pressure.[82–85] An augmentative treatment effect on reducing AHI was found in patients not responding to CPAP or MAD use alone.[82–84]

PRACTICE RECOMMENDATIONS
Indications

OAs in the form of MADs can be used as an alternative for patients of all OSA severities who are intolerant of CPAP or prefer an alternative therapy.[4]

Contraindications

Patients who are generally unsuitable for MAD treatment include edentulous patients and patients with inadequate number of sound teeth, severe periodontitis, and/or history of TMJ disease. There are exceptions, and MADs can sometimes be worn successfully by edentulous patients with good dentoalveolar ridges.[1] TSDs are not dependent on the dentition for retention and can be prescribed for edentulous or insufficiently dentate patients.

Appliance Selection

A plethora of designs is currently in use.[86] Based on current evidence, customized, titratable MADs are the preferred form of OAs.[4] TSDs can be used in MAD nonresponders who want OA therapy.

Clinical Follow-up

Trained dentists in sleep practice should follow-up patients using MADs to reduce dental side effects and occlusal changes.[4] Initial side effects are transient and reversible.[51,52] Close monitoring and coaching through the initial period may improve compliance.[35,50,51]

For initial comfort, mandibular advancement is 75% of maximum protrusion.[1] Clinical titration with an adaptation period increases the achievable protrusion and improves treatment response.[27]

Clinical titration should be followed by overnight PSG. Subjective feedback is not sufficient to determine the optimal setting of MAD. Post-PSG titration has been shown to improve MAD efficacy significantly.[4,28,75]

REFERENCES

1. Yow M, Lye EKW. Obstructive sleep apnea: orthodontic startegies to establish and maintain a patent airway. In: Krishnan V, Davidovitch Z, editors. Integrated clinical orthodontics. 1st edition. New Jersey (USA): Wiley-Blackwell Publishing Ltd; 2012. p. 214–39.
2. Sutherland K, Deane SA, Chan AS, et al. Comparative effects of two oral appliances on upper airway structure in obstructive sleep apnea. Sleep 2011; 34(4):469–77.
3. Deane SA, Cistulli PA, Ng AT, et al. Comparison of mandibular advancement splint and tongue stabilizing device in obstructive sleep apnea: a randomized controlled trial. Sleep 2009;32(5):648–53.
4. Ramar K, Dort LC, Katz SG, et al. Clinical practice guideline for the treatment of obstructive sleep apnea and snoring with oral appliance therapy: an update for 2015. J Clin Sleep Med 2015;11(7): 773–827.

5. Chang ET, Fernandez-Salvador C, Giambo J, et al. Tongue retaining devices for obstructive sleep apnea: a systematic review and meta-analysis. Am J Otolaryngol 2017;38(3):272–8.

6. Ishida M, Inoue Y, Suto Y, et al. Mechanism of action and therapeutic indication of prosthetic mandibular advancement in obstructive sleep apnea syndrome. Psychiatry Clin Neurosci 1998;52(2):227–9.

7. Ryan CF, Love LL, Peat D, et al. Mandibular advancement oral appliance therapy for obstructive sleep apnoea: effect on awake calibre of the velopharynx. Thorax 1999;54(11):972–7.

8. Chan AS, Lee RW, Srinivasan VK, et al. Nasopharyngoscopic evaluation of oral appliance therapy for obstructive sleep apnoea. Eur Respir J 2010; 35(4):836–42.

9. Chan AS, Sutherland K, Schwab RJ, et al. The effect of mandibular advancement on upper airway structure in obstructive sleep apnoea. Thorax 2010; 65(8):726–32.

10. Kato J, Isono S, Tanaka A, et al. Dose-dependent effects of mandibular advancement on pharyngeal mechanics and nocturnal oxygenation in patients with sleep-disordered breathing. Chest 2000; 117(4):1065–72.

11. Kuna ST, Woodson LC, Solanki DR, et al. Effect of progressive mandibular advancement on pharyngeal airway size in anesthetized adults. Anesthesiology 2008;109(4):605–12.

12. Choi JK, Hur YK, Lee JM, et al. Effects of mandibular advancement on upper airway dimension and collapsibility in patients with obstructive sleep apnea using dynamic upper airway imaging during sleep. Oral Surg Oral Med Oral Pathol Oral Radiol Endod 2010;109(5):712–9.

13. Brown EC, Cheng S, McKenzie DK, et al. Tongue and lateral upper airway movement with mandibular advancement. Sleep 2013;36(3):397–404.

14. Isono S, Tanaka A, Sho Y, et al. Advancement of the mandible improves velopharyngeal airway patency. J Appl Physiol (1985) 1995;79(6):2132–8.

15. Isono S, Tanaka A, Tagaito Y, et al. Pharyngeal patency in response to advancement of the mandible in obese anesthetized persons. Anesthesiology 1997;87(5):1055–62.

16. Pae EK, Lowe AA, Fleetham JA. A role of pharyngeal length in obstructive sleep apnea patients. Am J Orthod Dentofacial Orthop 1997;111(1):12–7.

17. Yoshida K. Effect of a prosthetic appliance for treatment of sleep apnea syndrome on masticatory and tongue muscle activity. J Prosthet Dent 1998;79(5): 537–44.

18. Johal A, Gill G, Ferman A, et al. The effect of mandibular advancement appliances on awake upper airway and masticatory muscle activity in patients with obstructive sleep apnoea. Clin Physiol Funct Imaging 2007;27(1):47–53.

19. Kurtulmus H, Cotert S, Bilgen C, et al. The effect of a mandibular advancement splint on electromyographic activity of the submental and masseter muscles in patients with obstructive sleep apnea. Int J Prosthodont 2009;22(6):586–93.

20. Malhotra A, Huang Y, Fogel RB, et al. The male predisposition to pharyngeal collapse: importance of airway length. Am J Respir Crit Care Med 2002; 166(10):1388–95.

21. Ng AT, Gotsopoulos H, Qian J, et al. Effect of oral appliance therapy on upper airway collapsibility in obstructive sleep apnea. Am J Respir Crit Care Med 2003;168(2):238–41.

22. Kushida CA, Morgenthaler TI, Littner MR, et al. Practice parameters for the treatment of snoring and Obstructive Sleep Apnea with oral appliances: an update for 2005. Sleep 2006;29(2):240–3.

23. Practice parameters for the treatment of snoring and obstructive sleep apnea with oral appliances. American Sleep Disorders Association. Sleep 1995;18(6): 511–3.

24. Sutherland K, Vanderveken OM, Tsuda H, et al. Oral appliance treatment for obstructive sleep apnea: an update. J Clin Sleep Med 2014;10(2):215–27.

25. Raphaelson MA, Alpher EJ, Bakker KW, et al. Oral appliance therapy for obstructive sleep apnea syndrome: progressive mandibular advancement during polysomnography. Cranio 1998;16(1):44–50.

26. Tsai WH, Vazquez JC, Oshima T, et al. Remotely controlled mandibular positioner predicts efficacy of oral appliances in sleep apnea. Am J Respir Crit Care Med 2004;170(4):366–70.

27. Gindre L, Gagnadoux F, Meslier N, et al. Mandibular advancement for obstructive sleep apnea: dose effect on apnea, long-term use and tolerance. Respiration 2008;76(4):386–92.

28. Almeida FR, Parker JA, Hodges JS, et al. Effect of a titration polysomnogram on treatment success with a mandibular repositioning appliance. J Clin Sleep Med 2009;5(3):198–204.

29. Aarab G, Lobbezoo F, Hamburger HL, et al. Effects of an oral appliance with different mandibular protrusion positions at a constant vertical dimension on obstructive sleep apnea. Clin Oral Investig 2010;14(3):339–45.

30. Dort L, Remmers J. A combination appliance for obstructive sleep apnea: the effectiveness of mandibular advancement and tongue retention. J Clin Sleep Med 2012;8(3):265–9.

31. Giles TL, Lasserson TJ, Smith BH, et al. Continuous positive airways pressure for obstructive sleep apnoea in adults. Cochrane Database Syst Rev 2006;(3):CD001106.

32. Lim J, Lasserson TJ, Fleetham J, et al. Oral appliances for obstructive sleep apnoea. Cochrane Database Syst Rev 2006;(1):CD004435.

33. Schwartz M, Acosta L, Hung YL, et al. Effects of CPAP and mandibular advancement device

treatment in obstructive sleep apnea patients: a systematic review and meta-analysis. Sleep Breath 2018;22(3):555–68.

34. Zhang M, Liu Y, Liu Y, et al. Effectiveness of oral appliances versus continuous positive airway pressure in treatment of OSA patients: an updated meta-analysis. Cranio 2018;1–18.

35. Dieltjens M, Verbruggen AE, Braem MJ, et al. Determinants of objective compliance during oral appliance therapy in patients with sleep-disordered breathing: a prospective clinical trial. JAMA Otolaryngol Head Neck Surg 2015;141(10):894–900.

36. Vanderveken OM, Dieltjens M, Wouters K, et al. Objective measurement of compliance during oral appliance therapy for sleep-disordered breathing. Thorax 2013;68(1):91–6.

37. Sutherland K, Phillips CL, Cistulli PA. Efficacy versus effectiveness in the treatment of obstructive sleep apnea: CPAP and oral appliances. J Dent Sleep Med 2015;2(4):175–81.

38. Lettieri CJ, Almeida FR, Cistulli PA, et al. Oral appliances for the treatment of obstructive sleep apnea-hypopnea syndrome and for concomitant sleep bruxism. In: MH K, T R, WC D, editors. Principles and practice of sleep medicine. 6th edition. Philadelphia: Elsevier; 2017. p. 1445–57.

39. Ahrens A, McGrath C, Hagg U. Subjective efficacy of oral appliance design features in the management of obstructive sleep apnea: a systematic review. Am J Orthod Dentofacial Orthop 2010;138(5):559–76.

40. Bratton DJ, Gaisl T, Schlatzer C, et al. Comparison of the effects of continuous positive airway pressure and mandibular advancement devices on sleepiness in patients with obstructive sleep apnoea: a network meta-analysis. Lancet Respir Med 2015;3(11):869–78.

41. Ng A, Gotsopoulos H, Darendeliler AM, et al. Oral appliance therapy for obstructive sleep apnea. Treat Respir Med 2005;4(6):409–22.

42. Blanco J, Zamarron C, Abeleira Pazos MT, et al. Prospective evaluation of an oral appliance in the treatment of obstructive sleep apnea syndrome. Sleep Breath 2005;9(1):20–5.

43. Gauthier L, Laberge L, Beaudry M, et al. Efficacy of two mandibular advancement appliances in the management of snoring and mild-moderate sleep apnea: a cross-over randomized study. Sleep Med 2009;10(3):329–36.

44. Kuhn E, Schwarz EI, Bratton DJ, et al. Effects of CPAP and mandibular advancement devices on health-related quality of life in OSA: a systematic review and meta-analysis. Chest 2017;151(4):786–94.

45. Bratton DJ, Gaisl T, Wons AM, et al. CPAP vs mandibular advancement devices and blood pressure in patients with obstructive sleep apnea: a systematic review and meta-analysis. Jama 2015;314(21):2280–93.

46. de Vries GE, Wijkstra PJ, Houwerzijl EJ, et al. Cardiovascular effects of oral appliance therapy in obstructive sleep apnea: a systematic review and meta-analysis. Sleep Med Rev 2018;40:55–68.

47. Van Haesendonck G, Dieltjens M, Kastoer C, et al. Cardiovascular benefits of oral appliance therapy in obstructive sleep apnea: a systematic review. J Dent Sleep Med 2015;2(1):9–14.

48. Anandam A, Patil M, Akinnusi M, et al. Cardiovascular mortality in obstructive sleep apnoea treated with continuous positive airway pressure or oral appliance: an observational study. Respirology 2013; 18(8):1184–90.

49. Attali V, Chaumereuil C, Arnulf I, et al. Predictors of long-term effectiveness to mandibular repositioning device treatment in obstructive sleep apnea patients after 1000 days. Sleep Med 2016;27-28:107–14.

50. Marklund M, Stenlund H, Franklin KA. Mandibular advancement devices in 630 men and women with obstructive sleep apnea and snoring: tolerability and predictors of treatment success. Chest 2004; 125(4):1270–8.

51. de Almeida FR, Lowe AA, Tsuiki S, et al. Long-term compliance and side effects of oral appliances used for the treatment of snoring and obstructive sleep apnea syndrome. J Clin Sleep Med 2005;1(2):143–52.

52. Ferguson KA, Cartwright R, Rogers R, et al. Oral appliances for snoring and obstructive sleep apnea: a review. Sleep 2006;29(2):244–62.

53. Araie T, Okuno K, Ono Minagi H, et al. Dental and skeletal changes associated with long-term oral appliance use for obstructive sleep apnea: a systematic review and meta-analysis. Sleep Med Rev 2018;41:161–72.

54. Pliska BT, Nam H, Chen H, et al. Obstructive sleep apnea and mandibular advancement splints: occlusal effects and progression of changes associated with a decade of treatment. J Clin Sleep Med 2014;10(12):1285–91.

55. Chen H, Lowe AA, de Almeida FR, et al. Three-dimensional computer-assisted study model analysis of long-term oral-appliance wear. Part 2. Side effects of oral appliances in obstructive sleep apnea patients. Am J Orthod Dentofacial Orthop 2008; 134(3):408–17.

56. Otsuka R, Almeida FR, Lowe AA. The effects of oral appliance therapy on occlusal function in patients with obstructive sleep apnea: a short-term prospective study. Am J Orthod Dentofacial Orthop 2007; 131(2):176–83.

57. Martinez-Gomis J, Willaert E, Nogues L, et al. Five years of sleep apnea treatment with a mandibular advancement device. Side effects and technical complications. Angle Orthod 2010;80(1):30–6.

58. Fransson AMC, Kowalczyk A, Isacsson G. A prospective 10-year follow-up dental cast study of patients with obstructive sleep apnoea/snoring who use a mandibular protruding device. Eur J Orthod 2017;39(5):502–8.

59. Alessandri-Bonetti G, D'Anto V, Stipa C, et al. Dentoskeletal effects of oral appliance wear in obstructive sleep apnoea and snoring patients. Eur J Orthod 2017;39(5):482–8.

60. Almeida FR, Lowe AA, Sung JO, et al. Long-term sequellae of oral appliance therapy in obstructive sleep apnea patients: Part 1. Cephalometric analysis. Am J Orthod Dentofacial Orthop 2006;129(2): 195–204.

61. Doff MH, Hoekema A, Pruim GJ, et al. Long-term oral-appliance therapy in obstructive sleep apnea: a cephalometric study of craniofacial changes. J Dent 2010;38(12):1010–8.

62. Eckert DJ, White DP, Jordan AS, et al. Defining phenotypic causes of obstructive sleep apnea. Identification of novel therapeutic targets. Am J Respir Crit Care Med 2013;188(8):996–1004.

63. Edwards BA, Eckert DJ, Jordan AS. Obstructive sleep apnoea pathogenesis from mild to severe: is it all the same? Respirology 2017;22(1):33–42.

64. Liu Y, Lowe AA, Fleetham JA, et al. Cephalometric and physiologic predictors of the efficacy of an adjustable oral appliance for treating obstructive sleep apnea. Am J Orthod Dentofacial Orthop 2001;120(6):639–47.

65. Okuno K, Pliska BT, Hamoda M, et al. Prediction of oral appliance treatment outcomes in obstructive sleep apnea: a systematic review. Sleep Med Rev 2016;30:25–33.

66. American Sleep Assocociation | sleep apnea oral appliances - research & treatments | 2018. Available at: https://www.sleepassociation.org/sleep-disorders/sleep-apnea/oral-appliance-for-sleep-apnea/. Accessed July 22, 2018.

67. Dieltjens M, Vanderveken OM, Heyning PH, et al. Current opinions and clinical practice in the titration of oral appliances in the treatment of sleep-disordered breathing. Sleep Med Rev 2012;16(2): 177–85.

68. Verbruggen AE, Vroegop AV, Dieltjens M, et al. Predicting Therapeutic Outcome of Mandibular Advancement Device Treatment in Obstructive Sleep Apnoea (PROMAD): study design and baseline characteristics. J Dent Sleep Med 2016;3(4): 119–38.

69. National Institutes of Health, United States National Library of Medicine, ClinicalTrials.gov. 2018. Available at: https://clinicaltrials.gov/ct2/show/record/NCT01532050. Accessed 26 July, 2018.

70. Alessandri-Bonetti G, Ippolito DR, Bartolucci ML, et al. Cephalometric predictors of treatment outcome with mandibular advancement devices in adult patients with obstructive sleep apnea: a systematic review. Korean J Orthod 2015;45(6):308–21.

71. Guarda-Nardini L, Manfredini D, Mion M, et al. Anatomically based outcome predictors of treatment for obstructive sleep apnea with intraoral splint devices: a systematic review of cephalometric studies. J Clin Sleep Med 2015;11(11):1327–34.

72. Vanderveken OM, Devolder A, Marklund M, et al. Comparison of a custom-made and a thermoplastic oral appliance for the treatment of mild sleep apnea. Am J Respir Crit Care Med 2008;178(2): 197–202.

73. Sasao Y, Nohara K, Okuno K, et al. Videoendoscopic diagnosis for predicting the response to oral appliance therapy in severe obstructive sleep apnea. Sleep Breath 2014;18(4):809–15.

74. Vroegop AV, Vanderveken OM, Dieltjens M, et al. Sleep endoscopy with simulation bite for prediction of oral appliance treatment outcome. J Sleep Res 2013;22(3):348–55.

75. Krishnan V, Collop NA, Scherr SC. An evaluation of a titration strategy for prescription of oral appliances for obstructive sleep apnea. Chest 2008;133(5): 1135–41.

76. Kuna ST, Giarraputo PC, Stanton DC, et al. Evaluation of an oral mandibular advancement titration appliance. Oral Surg Oral Med Oral Pathol Oral Radiol Endod 2006;101(5):593–603.

77. Petelle B, Vincent G, Gagnadoux F, et al. One-night mandibular advancement titration for obstructive sleep apnea syndrome: a pilot study. Am J Respir Crit Care Med 2002;165(8):1150–3.

78. Dort LC, Hadjuk E, Remmers JE. Mandibular advancement and obstructive sleep apnoea: a method for determining effective mandibular protrusion. Eur Respir J 2006;27(5):1003–9.

79. Remmers J, Charkhandeh S, Grosse J, et al. Remotely controlled mandibular protrusion during sleep predicts therapeutic success with oral appliances in patients with obstructive sleep apnea. Sleep 2013;36(10):1517–25, 1525A.

80. Sutherland K, Ngiam J, Cistulli PA. Performance of remotely controlled mandibular protrusion sleep studies for prediction of oral appliance treatment response. J Clin Sleep Med 2017;13(3):411–7.

81. Kastoer C, Dieltjens M, Oorts E, et al. The use of remotely controlled mandibular positioner as a predictive screening tool for mandibular advancement device therapy in patients with obstructive sleep apnea through single-night progressive titration of the mandible: a systematic review. J Clin Sleep Med 2016;12(10):1411–21.

82. Denbar MA. A case study involving the combination treatment of an oral appliance and auto-titrating CPAP unit. Sleep Breath 2002;6(3):125–8.

83. El-Solh AA, Moitheennazima B, Akinnusi ME, et al. Combined oral appliance and positive airway pressure therapy for obstructive sleep apnea: a pilot study. Sleep Breath 2011;15(2):203–8.

84. Liu HW, Chen YJ, Lai YC, et al. Combining MAD and CPAP as an effective strategy for treating patients with severe sleep apnea intolerant to high-pressure

PAP and unresponsive to MAD. PLoS One 2017; 12(10):e0187032.

85. de Vries GE, Doff MHJ, Hoekema A, et al. Continuous positive airway pressure and oral appliance hybrid therapy in obstructive sleep apnea: patient comfort, compliance, and preference: a pilot study. J Dent Sleep Med 2016;3(1):5–10.

86. Yow M. An overview of oral appliances and managing the airway in obstructive sleep apnea. Semin Orthod 2009;15(2):88–93.

Positional Therapy for Positional Obstructive Sleep Apnea

Mok Yingjuan, MBBS, MRCP[a],*,
Wong Hang Siang, MBBS, MRCP[a],
Tan Kah Leong Alvin, MBChB, MRCS[b],
Hsu Pon Poh, MBBS, MD[b]

KEYWORDS

- Positional sleep apnea • Positional therapy • Obstructive sleep apnea • Positional device

KEY POINTS

- A significant proportion of patients with obstructive sleep apnea (OSA) have positional OSA, where breathing abnormalities are reduced in a nonsupine sleeping position.
- Positional therapy is an attractive strategy for such patients, especially given the well-known challenges of standard continuous positive airway pressure (CPAP) treatment.
- The traditional "Tennis Ball Technique," however, failed to achieve widespread adoption due to poor patient tolerance and adherence.
- Recently, more sophisticated vibratory positional therapy devices have been developed with studies demonstrating efficacy and better patient tolerance compared with traditional methods.
- With the goal toward personalized treatment of OSA, positional therapy remains an active area of research. There are currently ongoing well-designed randomized controlled trials comparing the new positional devices with gold standard CPAP or as part of combination therapy.

INTRODUCTION

Positional obstructive sleep apnea (POSA) describes the condition in a group of patients with obstructive apneas and hypopneas that occur more frequently in certain sleep positions, notably in the supine position (**Fig. 1**). For these patients with POSA, positional therapy (PT) becomes an additional viable option for treatment. One of the earliest definitions of POSA was by Cartwright,[1] who proposed an overall apnea-hypopnea index (AHI) of more than 5 per hour and the supine apnea index to be at least twice that of the nonsupine apnea index. Since then, the criteria to diagnose POSA have been further modified with additional factors but retaining Cartwright's[1] criteria as the basic finding.

Depending on the diagnostic criteria used, patients with POSA make up 53.0% to 77.4% of those diagnosed with obstructive sleep apnea (OSA) following polysomnography (PSG).[2–5] Some Asian studies have demonstrated a higher prevalence of POSA. Teerapraipruk and colleagues[6] found the prevalence of POSA to be 67% in their study from Thailand. Three studies from South Korea showed that their prevalence of POSA was even higher at 74.7%,[7] 75.6%,[4] and 77.4%.[3]

Disclosure Statement: The authors have no conflict of interests to declare.
[a] Department of Respiratory and Critical Care Medicine, Changi General Hospital, 2 Simei Street 3, Singapore 529889; [b] Department of Otorhinolaryngology, Head and Neck Surgery, Changi General Hospital, 2 Simei Street 3, Singapore 529889
* Corresponding author.
E-mail address: ying_juan_mok@cgh.com.sg

Sleep Med Clin 14 (2019) 119–133
https://doi.org/10.1016/j.jsmc.2018.10.003

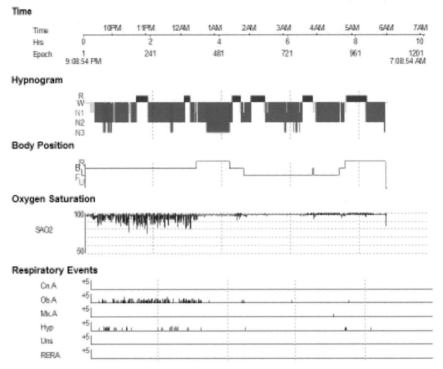

Fig. 1. Sleep study graphical summary of a subject with POSA.

TYPES OF CLASSIFICATION OF POSITIONAL OBSTRUCTIVE SLEEP APNEA

Presently, there are no universally accepted criteria used to diagnose POSA.

The most common criteria used to diagnose POSA are Cartwright's[1] rule of AHI more than 5 per hour and a supine apnea index being at least twice that of nonsupine apnea index, published in 1984.

In 2005, Mador and colleagues[5] modified the definition of POSA. Although he too defined POSA as a total AHI more than 5 per hour with a more than 50% reduction in the nonsupine AHI when compared with the supine AHI, he further classified patients with POSA into 2 groups: supine-predominant OSA (nonsupine AHI equal or more than 5 per hour) and supine-isolated OSA (nonsupine AHI <5 per hour), with at least 15 minutes of sleep in both positions.

More recently, in 2015, Frank and colleagues[8] proposed a new classification system called the Amsterdam Positional OSA Classification (APOC). The aim of this classification is to identify suitable candidates for PT in POSA. According to the APOC criteria, patients need to be diagnosed with OSA and must spend more than 10% of the total sleep time in both the best sleeping position (BSP) and worst sleeping position (WSP). The

patients with POSA are then classified into 3 categories as follows:

1. APOC I: BSP AHI less than 5
2. APOC II: BSP AHI in a lower OSA severity category
3. APOC III: Overall AHI of at least 40 and at least a 25% lower BSP AHI

Using the APOC helps to discriminate between the true patient with POSA who is cured with PT (APOC I), patients who can benefit from PT but are not cured (APOC II or III), and finally patients with nonpositional OSA. Patients in APOC II or III may benefit from combination therapies and may be eligible for lower continuous positive airway pressure (CPAP) requirements and less invasive surgery. This classification system has a better sensitivity, specificity, positive-predictive, and negative predictive value when compared with the classification of Cartwright[1] and Mador and colleagues.[5]

CLINICAL CHARACTERISTICS

Patients with POSA have certain distinctive clinical characteristics that differ from patients with non-positional OSA. Patients with POSA tend to be younger, have a lower body mass index (BMI), a smaller neck and waist circumference, as well as a lower prevalence of hypertension. They also score lower in Mallampati scores, Berlin questionnaires, STOP questionnaires, and Epworth Sleepiness Scale (ESS). When comparing polysomnographic data with patients with nonpositional OSA, patients with POSA sleep more in the nonsupine position, have a longer duration of total sleep time, better sleep efficiency, less wake after sleep onset, lower arousal index, lower AHI, and lower oxygen desaturation index (ODI). Patients with POSA have a higher proportion of stage 3 and rapid eye movement sleep when compared with their nonpositional counterparts.[1]

Mador and colleagues[5] showed that POSA was present in 49.5% of patients with mild OSA, 19.4% of patients with moderate OSA, and 6.5% of those with severe OSA. Mo and colleagues[7] showed in their Asian series that POSA was present in 87% of patients with mild OSA, 84.2% of patients with moderate OSA, and 43.1% of patients with severe OSA.

Studies also have demonstrated that patients with POSA have a lower snoring frequency, higher mean oxygen saturation, and higher nadir oxygen saturation when compared with patients with non-positional OSA.[6]

PATHOGENESIS

The pharyngeal critical closing pressure (PCrit) measures the pressure at which the upper airway collapses. A higher PCrit indicates that an airway is more collapsible. It has been demonstrated that PCrit is higher in the supine position when compared with the lateral position, indicating a higher collapsibility of the upper airway when supine.[9]

There are several explanations for the improvement in OSA in the nonsupine position when compared with supine.

Studies have shown that in the supine posture, retropalatal anteroposterior diameter and pharyngeal cross-sectional areas are reduced significantly.[10,11] This increases the likelihood of upper airway obstruction. Effects of gravity play a likely role in changing airway dimensions. Nonsupine posture reduces the directional effect of gravity on pharyngeal structures like the soft palate and tongue when compared with the supine posture. This is supported by a study on astronauts in weightlessness, which showed that AHI is lower in the absence of gravity compared with normal gravity.[12]

Lung volume has also been shown to affect the collapsibility of the upper airway, thereby influencing the pathogenesis of OSA. Stanchina and colleagues[13] showed that reducing lung volumes result in increased inspiratory airflow resistance and increased genioglossus muscle activation, causing the pharynx to be more collapsible. The effect of increased lung volume in decreasing upper airway collapsibility has been attributed to the former's effect on caudal trachea.[14] In the clinical setting, increasing BMI has an effect on reducing lung volume. Studies have shown that when patients change position to the supine posture, there is a reduction in total lung capacity, functional residual capacity, and vital capacity with a resultant increase in pulmonary flow-resistance and reduction in lung compliance.[15]

WHAT IS POSITIONAL THERAPY?

PT is defined as any technique used to avoid the worst sleeping position causing POSA. The worst sleeping position usually refers to the supine position.

The tennis ball technique (TBT) is the classic traditional PT in which a tennis ball–sized material is placed in a pocket stitched into the back of a patient's nightwear. TBT works by causing discomfort when sleeping on the back, forcing the patient to roll into a nonsupine position.

In 1984, a letter written by a patient's wife describing how she cured his snoring was first published in the journal *CHEST*. She sewed a pocket into the back of his T-shirt and inserted a hollow, lightweight plastic ball. By wearing this modified T-shirt during sleep, the patient stopped snoring and his daytime sleepiness resolved. Since then, various modifications of the TBT technique have been described over the years.

EFFICACY OF "TENNIS BALL TECHNIQUE" POSITIONAL THERAPY

De Vries and colleagues[16] evaluated the efficacy of TBT in a single-arm study of 53 patients, in whom 40 patients had a follow-up polysomnogram (PSG) (**Table 1**). The TBT mimickers included a commercial fabricated waistband as well as self-made constructions in the treatment of POSA. Overall AHI was found to decrease significantly after a median treatment time interval of 12 weeks (median AHI: 14.5–5.9/h, $P<.001$).

Jackson and colleagues[17] compared the use of a sleep position modification device (active group) to sleep hygiene advice (control group) in the treatment of POSA in a 4-week randomized controlled trial. Eighty-six subjects completed the trial, of which 47 were in the active group and 39 were in the control group. Both the supine sleep time and AHI were reduced significantly from baseline in the active group as compared with the control

Table 1
Trials using traditional positional therapy strategies

Author, Year	Design	Subjects and Sample Size, n	Intervention	Control	Follow-up Duration	Outcomes
de Vries et al,[16] 2015	Retrospective observational	Supine AHI 2x ≥ nonsupine AHI n = 40	TBT	NA	Median interval of 12 wk	AHI, compliance
Jackson et al,[17] 2015	Randomized controlled trial	Total AHI ≥10 supine AHI 2x ≥ nonsupine AHI n = 86	Sleep position modification device	Sleep hygiene	4 wk	Supine sleep time, AHI, quality of life, daytime sleepiness, mood, symptoms, neuropsychological measures, blood pressure
Zuberi et al,[18] 2004	Single arm	RDI >5/h n = 22	SONA pillow	NA	1 night without and 1 night with SONA pillow	RDI, SaO$_2$, snoring
Bidarian-Moniri et al,[19] 2015	Single arm	Mild to severe OSA n = 14	Pillow for prone positioning	NA	4 wk	AHI, ODI, supine sleep time, compliance
Loord et al,[20] 2007	Single arm	Supine AHI >15, lateral AHI <5 n = 23	"Positioner"	NA	3 mo	AHI, ESS, snoring
Berger et al,[21] 1997	Single arm	Total RDI ≥10; supine RDI 2x ≥ nonsupine RDI n = 13	TBT	NA	1 mo	Blood pressure

TBT vs CPAP

Jokic et al,[22] 1999	Randomized crossover	Lateral AHI <15/h; supine AHI 2x ≥ lateral AHI n = 13	Tennis ball in a backpack	CPAP	2 wk per arm	ESS, AHI, minimum SaO_2, sleep quality, MWT, psychometric test battery, mood scales, QOL, treatment preference
Skinner et al,[23] 2008	Randomized crossover trial	AHI >5/h; supine AHI 2x ≥AHI in other positions n = 20	Thoracic antisupine band	Nasal CPAP	1 mo per arm, with 1 wk washout	AHI, ESS, adherence, sleep quality and QOL, adverse effects
Permut et al,[24] 2010	Randomized crossover trial	Nonsupine AHI <5/h; supine AHI 2x ≥ nonsupine AHI n = 38	Zzoma Positional sleeper	CPAP	1 night per arm	AHI, total sleep time, supine sleep time, minimum SaO_2, treatment preference

Abbreviations: AHI, apnea-hypopnea index; CPAP, continuous positive airway pressure; ESS, Epworth sleepiness scale; MWT, maintenance of wakefulness; NA, not applicable; PT, positional therapy; QOL, quality of life; RDI, respiratory disturbance index; SaO_2, oxygen saturation; TBT, tennis ball technique.

group. However, no significant differences were seen in quality of life, daytime sleepiness, mood, neuropsychological measures, or blood pressure between both groups.

POSITIONAL THERAPY VERSUS CONTINUOUS POSITIVE AIRWAY PRESSURE

Jokic and colleagues[22] compared CPAP and PT in 13 patients with POSA in a randomized crossover trial. PT took the form of a soft ball placed in a backpack, a variation of the classic "TBT." Patients were randomized to either the PT or the CPAP intervention arm for 2 weeks before crossing over to the other arm for another 2 weeks. PT was shown to be effective in reducing sleep time in the supine position. PT was also able to decrease AHI, although a lower AHI was achieved with CPAP. In addition, minimum oxygen saturation was higher in the CPAP arm. Interestingly, no significant difference was found in terms of sleep architecture, daytime sleepiness, mood, or quality of life assessments. Of note, more patients preferred CPAP to PT (7 vs 4 respectively), with 2 having no preference.

Skinner and colleagues[23] conducted a similar study that compared 20 subjects with mild to moderate POSA in a randomized crossover trial. Subjects were randomized to a thoracic antisupine band as PT or nasal CPAP (nCPAP) for 1 month before crossing over to the opposite arm after a 1-week washout period. PT reduced mean AHI from 22.7 to 12.0 events per hour; however, more patients using nCPAP achieved treatment success compared with PT (16/18 vs 13/18, $P<.004$), defined as an AHI $\leq$10 events per hour. Mean AHI was also significantly lower in nCPAP compared with PT (4.9 vs 12.0, $P = .02$). Again, there was no significant difference in daytime sleepiness or quality of life indices between the 2 arms. However, as the primary outcome was AHI, the study may not be powered to detect differences in measures of symptoms and quality of life. It is noteworthy that subjective adherence was higher in PT and fewer side events were reported compared with nCPAP.

In another crossover trial, by Permut and colleagues[24] 38 patients with POSA were randomized to 1 night of sleep study with CPAP therapy followed by another night of sleep study with the Zzoma Positional Sleeper or vice versa. The Zzoma Positional Sleeper (**Fig. 2**) was made up of semi-rigid foam worn on the back like a backpack attached with a Velcro belt. PT using the Zzoma Positional Sleeper was shown to be as efficacious as CPAP at normalizing AHI to less than 5 events per hour (92% vs 97% of study subjects in the groups respectively, $P = .16$).

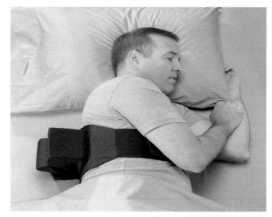

Fig. 2. Zzoma, a sleep position modification device that prevents a user from sleeping in the supine position. (*Courtesy of* ZzOMA, Bala Cynwyd, PA; with permission.)

OTHER POSITIONAL THERAPY TECHNIQUES

Techniques other than TBT have been studied over the years. Zuberi and colleagues[18] evaluated the efficacy of the SONA pillow in the treatment of 22 subjects with OSA. The SONA pillow was a specially designed inclined pillow that allowed one to place one's arm under the head while sleeping in a lateral recumbent position. In subjects with mild to moderate OSA, mean Respiratory Disturbance Index (RDI) was shown to decrease significantly from 17 events per hour to less than 5 events per hour while using the SONA Pillow ($P<.0001$). Bidarian-Moniri and colleagues[19] assessed the effectiveness of prone positioning through the combination of a mattress and pillow and again demonstrated a reduction in overall AHI in patients with OSA. Of note, however, both studies included all patients with OSA and no analysis was performed on treatment efficacy for patients with positional versus nonpositional OSA.

Loord and colleagues[20] conducted a trial in 2006 on 23 patients with POSA using a device called a "Positioner." It was a soft vest attached to a board placed under the pillow that prevents the patient from sleeping on the back; 18 patients completed the study. After 3 months of treatment, 61% of patients had a reduction in AHI to less than 10 per hour. Mean ESS however, decreased only from 12.3 to 10.2.

COMPLIANCE TO TRADITIONAL POSITIONAL THERAPY

Despite its apparent efficacy, PT has not been widely adopted in part due to the poor treatment adherence observed.

In a study by Oksenberg and colleagues,[25] TBT compliance was recorded at only 38% (19/50) at 6-month follow-up. In a longer term study by Bignold and colleagues,[26] fewer than 10% of patients were using their PT device after 30 months. In a more recent study in 2015 by de Vries and colleagues[16] on TBT, although short-term compliance appeared to be good (mean PT usage 7.2 hours per night), long-term compliance was again poor, with 65% of patients having stopped their PT usage after a mean of 13 months. Of note, PT compliance was measured with self-reported questionnaires in the studies.

In 2012, Heinzer and colleagues[27] objectively measured treatment compliance in 16 subjects at 3 months with a built-in actigraphy within a TBT device. Actigraphy recordings demonstrated that the patients used the device 73.7% ± 29.3% of the nights (range 9%–100%) for an average of 8.0 ± 2.0 hours per night (range 3.8–10.6 hours). Ten patients used PT for more than 80% of the nights with 13 using more than 60% of the nights.

LIMITATIONS OF POSITIONAL THERAPY TRIALS

Most studies performed with the traditional PT have significant limitations. Many are underpowered, have different definitions of POSA, and different outcome measures. Treatment adherence was mostly measured through subjective reporting by patients, potentially leading to reporting bias. There is also a lack of trials evaluating clinical outcomes with PT therapy in the treatment of POSA. A study by Berger and colleagues[21] in 1997 had been the only trial assessing the effect of TBT on blood pressure as the primary outcome.

NEW POSITIONAL THERAPY DEVICES

Recent technological advances have renewed interest in PT for the treatment of POSA. In the past few years, more sophisticated PT devices have been developed and they appeared to be better than the traditional PT strategies. The new devices are the Night Shift,[28] Sleep Position Trainer (SPT),[29] and BuzzPOD.[30] The small Night Shift device (**Fig. 3**) is worn at the back of the neck with a latex-free silicone rubber strap that is secured using a magnetic clasp. The SPT (**Fig. 4**) and BuzzPOD (**Fig. 5**) are small devices placed on the sternum or chest and secured in place with a chest strap. An in-built accelerometer in these devices ascertains the neck position (Night Shift) or body position (SPT and BuzzPOD) of the

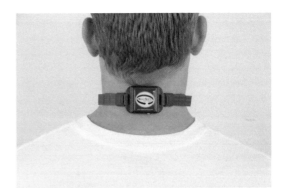

Fig. 3. Night Shift, a neck-worn vibrating PT device. (*Courtesy of* Night Shift, Carlsbad, CA; with permission.)

user during sleep. When a supine position is detected, the devices vibrate with increasing intensity until the patient changes to a nonsupine position. Of the 3 devices, the Night Shift is currently the only one approved by the US Food and Drug Administration for the treatment POSA.

EFFICACY OF THE NEW POSITIONAL THERAPY DEVICES

In 2011, Bignold and colleagues[30] first evaluated a novel position monitoring device with an in-built supine avoidance vibratory alarm in a randomized controlled crossover trial of 15 patients with POSA (**Table 2**). Subjects were randomized to the vibratory positional therapy device or no treatment for 1 week before crossing over to opposite arm after a 1-week washout period. This device significantly reduced mean percentage of supine sleep time and mean AHI (25–13.7 events per hour, $P = .03$).

In 2013, van Maanen and colleagues[29] demonstrated the ability of the SPT device to significantly reduce median percentage of supine sleeping time and median AHI in 31 subjects with POSA after 4 weeks of treatment in a single-arm study. ESS was found to be significantly decreased and the Functional Outcomes of Sleep Questionnaire (FOSQ) scores improved significantly.

In a more recent randomized controlled trial in 2017, Laub and colleagues[31] compared the use of the SPT device (52 subjects) versus no treatment (49 subjects) in patients with POSA. The reduction in mean total AHI with SPT was shown to remain significant after 6 months. Daytime sleepiness also improved after 6 months of SPT treatment.

The evaluation of a small vibrating neck-worn apparatus was first performed by van Maanen and colleagues[32] in 2012 on 30 patients with POSA. Mean AHI was decreased from 27.7 ± 2.4

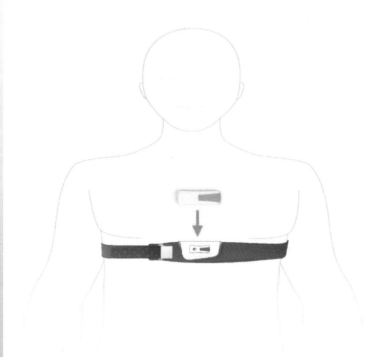

Fig. 4. NightBalance Sleep Position Trainer, a chest-worn vibratory PT device. (*Courtesy of* Night Balance BV, Delft, Netherlands; with permission.)

per hour to 12.8 ± 2.2 per hour (*P*<.05). Subsequently in 2014, Levendowski at al[28] demonstrated that after a 4-week use of the neck-worn Night Shift PT device, the overall AHI of 30 patients with POSA decreased from 24.7 ± 14.7 per hour to 7.5 ± 7.7 per hour (*P*<.00001). This study also showed a significant improvement in sleep architecture and Patient Health Questionnaire-9 depression score (*P* = .027).

NEW POSITIONAL THERAPIES VERSUS TENNIS BALL TECHNIQUE

In 2015, Eijsvogel and colleagues[33] compared the efficacy of the SPT device with that of the

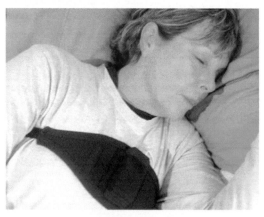

Fig. 5. BuzzPod, a chest-worn vibratory PT device. (*Courtesy of* BuzzPod, Victoria, Australia; with permission.)

traditional TBT in patients with POSA. Both therapies (29 patients in SPT arm and 26 patients in TBT arm) reduced supine sleep position to a median of 0% (minimum-maximum: SPT 0.0% to 67%, TBT 0.0% to 38.9%). Treatment success was defined as AHI less than 5 per hour and appeared to be higher in the SPT group (68.0%) compared with the TBT group (42.9%) although this was not statistically significant. Greater improvements were seen in the SPT arm compared with the TBT arm with regard to sleep quality, total QSQ (Quebec Sleep Questionnaire) scores, the QSQ domains of nocturnal symptoms, and social interactions.

NEW POSITIONAL THERAPY DEVICES VERSUS CONTINUOUS POSITIVE AIRWAY PRESSURE

To date, there are no published data from a randomized controlled trial comparing the new vibratory PT devices with the gold standard CPAP in the treatment of POSA. Three crossover randomized controlled trials are currently ongoing to compare the efficacy of these new vibratory PT devices to CPAP in POSA patients (**Table 3**).

The POSAtive study (ClinicalTrials.gov: NCT03061071)[34] is a multicenter trial in Europe that compares the Nightbalance SPT with autoCPAP. A total of 120 subjects with POSA will be randomized to either treatment for 6 weeks, before crossing over to the alternative treatment arm. The primary outcomes to be studied are treatment adherence and AHI.

Table 2
Trials using new vibratory positional therapy devices

Author, Year	Design	Subjects and Sample Size, n	Intervention	Control	Follow-up Duration	Outcomes
Levendowski et al,[28] 2014	Single arm	Overall AHI ≥5; overall AHI 1.5x ≥ nonsupine AHI n = 30	Neck-worn vibrating device (Night Shift)	NA	4 wk	AHI, % time SaO₂<90%, depression score, sleep architecture
van Maanen et al,[29] 2013	Single arm	supine AHI 2x ≥ nonsupine AHI n = 36	SPT	NA	1 mo	AHI, sleep efficiency, ESS, functional outcomes of sleep questionnaire, compliance
Bignold et al,[30] 2011	Randomized controlled crossover trial	Total AHI >5/h; nonsupine AHI <15/h; supine AHI 2x ≥ nonsupine AHI n = 15	A position monitoring and supine alarm device	No treatment	1 wk per arm with 1 wk washout	AHI, snoring frequency, supine sleep time
Laub et al,[31] 2017	Randomized controlled trial	Supine AHI 2x ≥ nonsupine AHI; supine AHI ≥10 per h; nonsupine AHI <10 per h n = 101	SPT	No treatment	2 mo and 6 mo	Supine sleep time, AHI, ESS, compliance
van Maanen et al,[32] 2012	Single arm	AHI >5; supine AHI 2x ≥ nonsupine AHI n = 30	Neck-worn vibrating device	NA	1 night with no device, 1 night with device on, 1 night with device off	AHI, supine sleep time
Eijsvogel et al,[33] 2015	Prospective randomized trial	Nonsupine AHI <10/h; supine AHI 2x ≥ nonsupine AHI n = 55	SPT	TBT	1 mo	Supine sleep time, AHI, ESS, sleep quality, QSQ, compliance

Abbreviations: AHI, apnea-hypopnea index; ESS, Epworth sleepiness scale; NA, not applicable; PT, positional therapy; QSQ, Quebec sleep questionnaire; SaO₂, oxygen saturation; SPT, sleep position trainer; TBT, tennis ball technique.

Table 3
Comparing the new positional therapy devices and other obstructive sleep apnea treatment modalities

Author, Year	Design	Subjects and Sample Size, n	Intervention A	Intervention B	Follow-up Duration	Outcomes
ClinicalTrials.gov Identifier: NCT03061071,[34] Ongoing	Multicenter randomized crossover trial	Total AHI >15, or 10< AHI <15 with ESS >10; supine AHI 2x ≥ nonsupine AHI, nonsupine AHI <10 (<5 in mild patients) n = 200	Sleep Position Trainer	Automated CPAP	6 wk	Primary outcomes: adherence, AHI Secondary outcomes: ESS, FOSQ, SF36, patient satisfaction, sleep parameters, mean disease alleviation
ACTRN12613001242718,[35] Ongoing	Randomized crossover trial	ESS: ≥8; AHI >10, nonsupine AHI <10; Supine AHI 2x ≥ nonsupine AHI n = 140	BuzzPOD supine avoidance device	CPAP	8 wk	Primary outcomes: Change in ESS Secondary outcomes: AHI, snoring, sleep quality, QOL, adherence, patient and partner satisfaction
ClinicalTrials.gov Identifier: NCT03125512,[40] Ongoing	Randomized crossover trial	ESS: ≥10; AHI >10, nonsupine AHI <10; Supine AHI 2x ≥nonsupine AHI n = 40	Night Shift Positional Device	Automated CPAP	8 wk	Primary outcomes: Difference in ESS Secondary outcomes: Treatment preference, AHI, FOSQ, SF36, sleep quality, mood and QOL questionnaires
Comparing the new PT devices and Oral Appliance						
Benoist et al,[36] 2017	Prospective multicenter randomized controlled trial	AHI ≥ 5 ≤ 30; Supine AHI 2x ≥ nonsupine AHI n = 99	SPT	Oral appliance therapy	3 mo	Primary outcome: AHI Secondary outcomes: ODI, sleepiness, sleep quality, adherence, mean disease alleviation, QOL, side effects

Study	Design	n / Population	Intervention	Comparator	Duration	Outcomes
Maurits et al,[41] 2018	(12-mo follow-up of the above trial)	n = 99	SPT	Oral appliance therapy	12 mo	
The new PT devices as part of combination therapy						
Dieltjens et al,[37] 2015	Randomized crossover trial	n = 20	SPT	Oral mandibular device + SPT	1 night per arm	Primary outcome: AHI Secondary outcomes: supine sleeping time, patient preference, sleep study parameters
Benoist et al,[38] 2017	Prospective single-arm study	Subjects with residual positional OSA after surgery n = 33	Sleep Position Trainer	NA	3 mo	AHI, sleep position parameters, daytime sleepiness, compliance, mean disease alleviation, QOL
ClinicalTrials.gov NCT02553902,[39] Ongoing	Multicenter randomized clinical trial	Moderate positional OSA (15< AHI <30); supine AHI 2x ≥ nonsupine AHI n = 200	Sleep Position Trainer + MAD	CPAP	3, 6, and 12 mo	AHI, compliance, QOL, economic evaluation, cardiovascular parameters

Abbreviations: AHI, apnea-hypopnea index; CPAP, continuous positive airway pressure; ESS, Epworth sleepiness scale; FOSQ, functional outcomes of sleep questionnaire; NA, not applicable; ODI, oxygen desaturation index; PT, positional therapy; QOL, quality of life; SF36, 36-item short form health survey; SPT, sleep position trainer.

The second study (ClinicalTrials.gov: NCT03125512) is a crossover randomized controlled trial currently being conducted in Singapore, a multiethnic Asian country. This study compares the Night Shift PT device with autoC-PAP. A total of 40 subjects with POSA and significant daytime sleepiness (defined as an ESS $\geq$10) will be randomized to either treatment for 8 weeks before crossing over to the alternative arm with a 1-week washout period in-between. The primary outcome is the difference in daytime sleepiness between the 2 arms after 8 weeks of device use. We look forward to its results, as studies on the new PT devices have mostly been conducted in the white population.

The SUPA OSA Trial[35] is a multicenter randomized controlled trial being conducted in South Australia that compares the BuzzPOD device with CPAP in the treatment of POSA. Due to recruitment challenges in meeting the original target sample size of 280 patients, the study was redesigned to become a crossover trial with a revised target sample size of 140. Subjects with POSA and ESS score $\geq$8 will be randomized to either treatment for 8 weeks, before crossing over to the opposite treatment arm after a 1 week washout interval. The primary outcome is the change in daytime sleepiness.

NEW POSITIONAL THERAPY DEVICES VERSUS ORAL APPLIANCE THERAPY

Benoist and colleagues[36] recently published their results from a multicenter, prospective randomized controlled trial that compared the SPT with oral appliance therapy (OAT) for the treatment of POSA. In this study, 99 subjects with mild to moderate POSA were randomized to either SPT or OAT for 3 months and 81 subjects completed the study. In the intention-to-treat (ITT) analysis, both SPT and OAT decreased the median AHI (SPT: 13.0–7.0/h, OAT: 11.7–9.1/h) and there were no significant differences between the 2 groups at 3 months (P = .535). Similarly, no between-group difference in AHI reduction at 3 months was observed in the per-protocol analysis. Mean adherence on per-protocol analysis was comparable between both interventions (SPT: 89.3% vs OAT: 81.3%) although adjusted adherence on ITT analysis was higher in SPT compared with OAT (SPT: 88.4%, OAT: 60.5%). There was no significant difference in mean disease alleviation. The investigators concluded that SPT and OAT were equivalent in the treatment of mild to moderate POSA with regard to AHI reduction. Of note, the OAT group reported a higher frequency of adverse events (n = 26, 26.8%) compared with the SPT group (n = 13, 13.4%). In addition, 15 of the 18 subjects who dropped out of the study came from the OAT intervention arm.

NEW POSITIONAL THERAPY DEVICES AS PART OF COMBINATION THERAPY

Dieltjens and colleagues[37] conducted a crossover randomized controlled trial to evaluate the efficacy of the SPT device in combination with mandibular advancement device (MAD) for the treatment of residual POSA. This study included patients with OSA who had undergone treatment with mandibular advancement device, but demonstrated residual POSA on PSG. The inclusion criteria were a residual AHI between 5 and 50 per hour and a supine AHI $\geq$2x nonsupine AHI. Of note, another inclusion criterion was the amount of supine sleeping time must be at least 20% of total sleep time during the PSG while wearing the MAD. Twenty patients with residual OSA on MAD were randomized to either SPT only or combination therapy with both MAD and SPT for a single-night PSG. They subsequently cross over to the opposite arm for a second PSG. The results demonstrated that the combination of MAD and SPT was most effective in reducing median overall AHI (from 20.9/h to 5.5/h) although individually, MAD and SPT were also able to significantly reduce AHI from baseline (to 11.6/h and 12.8/h, respectively). With combination therapy, 95% of subjects achieved treatment success, defined as a minimum of 50% or more reduction in overall AHI. Seven of 15 subjects indicated preference for combination therapy. Further studies would be required to evaluate longer term efficacy and treatment adherence.

Benoist and colleagues[38] evaluated the role of positional therapy in subjects with residual POSA despite surgery. In a prospective single-arm study, 33 subjects with residual POSA after upper airway surgery were treated with the SPT for 3 months. Of note, 76% of the subjects had failed CPAP treatment and 48.5% had failed oral appliance therapy before study participation. A decrease in overall AHI of at least 50% was deemed to be a positive treatment response, and treatment success was achieved if overall AHI was reduced to less than 5 per hour. The results revealed that PT was able to further decrease the median postoperative AHI from 18.3 per hour to 12.5 per hour and the ESS from 10 to 7 after 3 months; 37.5% (n = 12) and 31.3% (n = 10) of the subjects had treatment response and treatment success, respectively. Mean disease alleviation (MDA) with PT was shown to be 41.3%, thereby increasing the overall MDA to 65.6% when combined with surgery.

Nevertheless, 20 subjects remained as nonresponders and further research is warranted to identify predictors of treatment response to PT. When compared with responders, nonresponders were found to have a higher AHI, supine AHI, nonsupine AHI, and ODI. The investigators hypothesized that one of the reasons for nonresponse to PT treatment could be the disparity in head position when the trunk is lateral, given that the positional device is worn on the chest.

There is currently an ongoing multicenter randomized controlled trial in Europe (ClinicalTrials.gov NCT02553902)[39] that aims to compare combination therapy with the gold standard CPAP for the treatment of POSA. A total of 200 patients with moderate POSA will be randomized to either the gold standard CPAP or combination therapy comprising both the SPT and mandibular advancement device. The study will evaluate treatment efficacy, adherence, quality of life indices, cardiovascular parameters, and cost-effectiveness.

COMPLIANCE WITH THE NEW POSITIONAL THERAPY DEVICES

Treatment adherence with the new vibratory positional devices has generally appeared to be high, possibly due to enhanced patient comfort with their petite design. In a study by Van Maanen and colleagues[29] using the Sleep Position Trainer, a treatment adherence rate of as high as 92.7% was reported at 1 month. Treatment adherence was defined as more than 4 hours of device use per day during 7 days a week. In the 2 studies by Benoist and colleagues[36,38] mentioned previously, treatment adherence was 89.3%[36] and 89.0%,[38] respectively, at 3 months, when defined as mean daily device use of at least 4 hours per night for a minimum of 5 days a week.

Van Maanen and colleagues[42] were the first to report the long-term compliance rate of the SPT device in a multicenter prospective cohort study of 145 subjects. At 6 months, 106 subjects had available device data and 71.2% achieved regular use of their device, defined as more than 4 hours. Over 5 days per week, 64.4% of subjects used more than 4 hours of their device/night across all nights. Subsequently, in an even longer follow-up study of 12 months by de Ruiter and colleagues,[41] 29 patients assigned SPT who completed follow-up were found to have an average device use per night of 5.2 hours; 82% used their PT device for more than 4 hours over 7 days per week.

Overall, the results of these studies are promising, although they were mainly performed with the SPT device. It remains to be seen if comparable results can be achieved with other new vibratory PT devices.

SUMMARY AND FUTURE DIRECTIONS

Significant progress in positional therapy has been made with the recent advent of new vibratory PT devices. Studies have demonstrated that these new PT devices are efficacious in reducing overall AHI and better tolerated by patients. Short-term and long-term treatment adherence also appears to be markedly higher compared with traditional positional therapy methods.

Nevertheless, more research is required to determine if the new PT devices can be offered as first-line treatment to patients with positional OSA. Most of the latest evidence has been limited to a single PT device and further studies would be necessary to evaluate if the results are generalizable to all devices. Most studies have also been conducted in the Caucasian population, and these positive results would need to be replicated in other ethnic groups in which genetic, anatomic, and societal traits are likely to differ.

In addition, there is currently a lack of high-quality evidence comparing these new devices with the gold standard CPAP in the treatment of positional OSA. Three randomized controlled trials are under way to address this important clinical question and we look forward to their results. PT as part of combination therapy in the personalized treatment of OSA is also another active area of research. It is hoped that these latest advances in positional therapy may offer an equivalent treatment alternative to many patients with positional OSA who are struggling with CPAP.

REFERENCES

1. Cartwright RD. Effect of sleep position on sleep apnea severity. Sleep 1984;7(2):110–4.
2. Oulhaj A, Al Dhaheri S, Su BB, et al. Discriminating between positional and non-positional obstructive sleep apnea using some clinical characteristics. Sleep Breath 2017;21(4):877–84.
3. Kim KT, Cho YW, Kim DE, et al. Two subtypes of positional obstructive sleep apnea: supine-predominant and supine-isolated. Clin Neurophysiol 2016;127(1):565–70.
4. Lee SA, Paek JH, Chung YS, et al. Clinical features in patients with positional obstructive sleep apnea according to its subtypes. Sleep Breath 2017; 21(1):109–17.
5. Mador MJ, Kufel TJ, Magalang UJ, et al. Prevalence of positional sleep apnea in patients undergoing polysomnography. Chest 2005;128(4):2130–7.

6. Teerapraipruk B, Chirakalwasan N, Simon R, et al. Clinical and polysomnographic data of positional sleep apnea and its predictors. Sleep Breath 2012; 16(4):1167–72.

7. Mo JH, Lee CH, Rhee CS, et al. Positional dependency in Asian patients with obstructive sleep apnea and its implication for hypertension. Arch Otolaryngol Head Neck Surg 2011;137(8):786–90.

8. Frank MH, Ravesloot MJ, van Maanen JP, et al. Positional OSA part 1: towards a clinical classification system for position-dependent obstructive sleep apnoea. Sleep Breath 2015;19(2):473–80.

9. Penzel T, Moller M, Becker HF, et al. Effect of sleep position and sleep stage on the collapsibility of the upper airways in patients with sleep apnea. Sleep 2001;24(1):90–5.

10. Yildirim N, Fitzpatrick MF, Whyte KF, et al. The effect of posture on upper airway dimensions in normal subjects and in patients with the sleep apnea/hypopnea syndrome. Am Rev Respir Dis 1991;144(4): 845–7.

11. Jan MA, Marshall I, Douglas NJ. Effect of posture on upper airway dimensions in normal human. Am J Respir Crit Care Med 1994;149(1):145–8.

12. Elliott AR, Shea SA, Dijk DJ, et al. Microgravity reduces sleep-disordered breathing in humans. Am J Respir Crit Care Med 2001;164(3):478–85.

13. Stanchina ML, Malhotra A, Fogel RB, et al. The influence of lung volume on pharyngeal mechanics, collapsibility, and genioglossus muscle activation during sleep. Sleep 2003;26(7):851–6.

14. Kairaitis K, Byth K, Parikh R, et al. Tracheal traction effects on upper airway patency in rabbits: the role of tissue pressure. Sleep 2007;30(2):179–86.

15. Behrakis PK, Baydur A, Jaeger MJ, et al. Lung mechanics in sitting and horizontal body positions. Chest 1983;83(4):643–6.

16. de Vries GE, Hoekema A, Doff MH, et al. Usage of positional therapy in adults with obstructive sleep apnea. J Clin Sleep Med 2015;11(2):131–7.

17. Jackson M, Collins A, Berlowitz D, et al. Efficacy of sleep position modification to treat positional obstructive sleep apnea. Sleep Med 2015;16(4): 545–52.

18. Zuberi NA, Rekab K, Nguyen HV. Sleep apnea avoidance pillow effects on obstructive sleep apnea syndrome and snoring. Sleep Breath 2004;8(4): 201–7.

19. Bidarian-Moniri A, Nilsson M, Attia J, et al. Mattress and pillow for prone positioning for treatment of obstructive sleep apnoea. Acta Otolaryngol 2015; 135(3):271–6.

20. Loord H, Hultcrantz E. Positioner–a method for preventing sleep apnea. Acta Otolaryngol 2007; 127(8):861–8.

21. Berger M, Oksenberg A, Silverberg DS, et al. Avoiding the supine position during sleep lowers 24 h blood pressure in obstructive sleep apnea (OSA) patients. J Hum Hypertens 1997;11(10):657–64.

22. Jokic R, Klimaszewski A, Crossley M, et al. Positional treatment vs continuous positive airway pressure in patients with positional obstructive sleep apnea syndrome. Chest 1999;115(3):771–81.

23. Skinner MA, Kingshott RN, Filsell S, et al. Efficacy of the 'tennis ball technique' versus nCPAP in the management of position-dependent obstructive sleep apnoea syndrome. Respirology 2008;13(5): 708–15.

24. Permut I, Diaz-Abad M, Chatila W, et al. Comparison of positional therapy to CPAP in patients with positional obstructive sleep apnea. J Clin Sleep Med 2010;6(3):238–43.

25. Oksenberg A, Silverberg D, Offenbach D, et al. Positional therapy for obstructive sleep apnea patients: a 6-month follow-up study. Laryngoscope 2006; 116(11):1995–2000.

26. Bignold JJ, Deans-Costi G, Goldsworthy MR, et al. Poor long-term patient compliance with the tennis ball technique for treating positional obstructive sleep apnea. J Clin Sleep Med 2009;5(5):428–30.

27. Heinzer RC, Pellaton C, Rey V, et al. Positional therapy for obstructive sleep apnea: an objective measurement of patients' usage and efficacy at home. Sleep Med 2012;13(4):425–8.

28. Levendowski DJ, Seagraves S, Popovic D, et al. Assessment of a neck-based treatment and monitoring device for positional obstructive sleep apnea. J Clin Sleep Med 2014;10(8):863–71.

29. van Maanen JP, Meester KA, Dun LN, et al. The sleep position trainer: a new treatment for positional obstructive sleep apnoea. Sleep Breath 2013;17(2): 771–9.

30. Bignold JJ, Mercer JD, Antic NA, et al. Accurate position monitoring and improved supine-dependent obstructive sleep apnea with a new position recording and supine avoidance device. J Clin Sleep Med 2011;7(4):376–83.

31. Laub RR, Tonnesen P, Jennum PJ. A Sleep Position Trainer for positional sleep apnea: a randomized, controlled trial. J Sleep Res 2017;26(5):641–50.

32. van Maanen JP, Richard W, Van Kesteren ER, et al. Evaluation of a new simple treatment for positional sleep apnoea patients. J Sleep Res 2012;21(3): 322–9.

33. Eijsvogel MM, Ubbink R, Dekker J, et al. Sleep position trainer versus tennis ball technique in positional obstructive sleep apnea syndrome. J Clin Sleep Med 2015;11(2):139–47.

34. ClinicalTrials.gov. Bethesda (MD): National Library of Medicine (US). 2000 Feb 29-. Identifier NCT03061071, The POSAtive Study: Study for the Treatment of Positional Obstructive Sleep Apnea. 2017. Available at: https://www.clinicaltrials.gov/ct2/

show/NCT03061071?cond=positional+obstructive+sleep+apnea&rank=4. Accessed July 1, 2018.

35. Australian New Zealand Clinical Trials Registry: Sydney (NSW): NHMRC Clinical Trials Centre, University of Sydney (Australia); 2005-. Identifier. ACTRN1 2613001242718. Does a supine-avoidance device achieve a similar reduction in sleepiness as usual CPAP treatment in patients with supine-predominant obstructive sleep apnoea? 2013. Available at: http://www.anzctr.org.au/TrialSearch.aspx?searchTxt=SUPA+OSA&isBasic=True. Accessed July 1, 2018.

36. Benoist L, de Ruiter M, de Lange J, et al. A randomized, controlled trial of positional therapy versus oral appliance therapy for position-dependent sleep apnea. Sleep Med 2017;34: 109–17.

37. Dieltjens M, Vroegop AV, Verbruggen AE, et al. A promising concept of combination therapy for positional obstructive sleep apnea. Sleep Breath 2015; 19(2):637–44.

38. Benoist LBL, Verhagen M, Torensma B, et al. Positional therapy in patients with residual positional obstructive sleep apnea after upper airway surgery. Sleep Breath 2017;21(2):279–88.

39. ClinicalTrials.gov. Bethesda (MD):National Library of Medicine (US). 2000 Feb 29-. Identifier NCT02553902, Economic evaluation of treatment modalities for position dependent obstructive sleep apnea; 2015. Available at: https://www.clinicaltrials.gov/ct2/show/NCT02553902?term=NCT02553902&rank=1. Accessed July 1, 2018.

40. ClinicalTrials.gov. Bethesda (MD): National Library of Medicine (US). 2000 Feb 29-. Identifier NCT03125512, Positional Therapy Versus CPAP for Positional OSA;2017. Available at: https://www.clinicaltrials.gov/ct2/show/NCT03125512?cond=positional+obstructive+sleep+apnea&rank=5. Accessed July 1, 2018.

41. de Ruiter MHT, Benoist LBL, de Vries N, et al. Durability of treatment effects of the Sleep Position Trainer versus oral appliance therapy in positional OSA: 12-month follow-up of a randomized controlled trial. Sleep Breath 2018;22(2):441–50.

42. van Maanen JP, de Vries N. Long-term effectiveness and compliance of positional therapy with the sleep position trainer in the treatment of positional obstructive sleep apnea syndrome. Sleep 2014;37(7): 1209–15.

Myofunctional Therapy
Role in Pediatric OSA

Yu-Shu Huang, MD, PhD[a,1], Shih-Chieh Hsu, MD[b,1], Christian Guilleminault, DM, MD, DBiol[c], Li-Chuan Chuang, DDS, MS[d,e],*

KEYWORDS

- Obstructive sleep apnea syndrome • Myofunctional therapy • Functional oral appliance
- Lateral cephalometric • Polysomnography

KEY POINTS

- Myofunctional therapy (MFT) has been reported to be an alternative treatment to obstructive sleep apnea (OSA), but compliance and long-term outcome in the children were considered as an issue.
- Compliance is a major problem of MFT, and MFT will have to take into consideration the absolute need to have continuous parental involvement in the procedure for pediatric OSA.
- Passive MFT gives more improved measurements and better compliance, but potential negative effects of device on other jaw will have to be continuously evaluated.

INTRODUCTION

Obstructive sleep apnea (OSA) is a common and serious disorder that affects the health of the general public.[1] The pathophysiology of OSA is complex. Most cyclical and cessations in sleep-disordered breathing events are driven by anomalies in both anatomic and neurochemical control of upper airway and/or chest wall respiratory musculature.[2] Therefore, several medical and surgical treatment modalities exist as treatment for OSA.[3–5] The causes of OSA are different between adult and children. Guilleminault and colleagues[6,7] published a review of 50 pediatric patients, which demonstrated that the clinical features of pediatric OSA were different from that of adults in 1981. Among the types of pediatric sleep-disordered breathing (SDB), OSA has the highest prevalence[8] but its pathophysiology continues to be unclear. Such as adenotonsillar

Funding source Study supported by Chang Gung Memorial Hospital, Taoyuan, Taiwan grant #: CMRPG 3H0781 to Y.-S. Huang and S.C. Hsu.

Financial Disclosure: None of the authors has financial interest relevant to this article to disclose.

Conflict of Interest: None of the authors has conflict of interest to disclose.

All authors approved the final article and agree to be accountable for all aspects of the work.

Approval of the protocol by the institutional review board of CGMH (201601757A3).

Conflict of Interest: All authors declare no conflicts of interest.

Author Contributions: Study conception and design: Y.S. Huang, and C Guilleminault. Acquisition of data: L.C. Chuang, and Y.S. Huang. Analysis and interpretation of cephalometric data: L.C. Chuang. Drafting of manuscript: Y.S. Huang, C Guilleminault and L.C. Chuang.

[a] Department of Child Psychiatry and Sleep Center, Chang Gung Memorial Hospital and College of Medicine, No. 5, Fuxing Street, Guishan, Taoyuan 333, Taiwan; [b] Department of Psychiatry and Sleep Center, Chang Gung Memorial Hospital and College of Medicine, No. 5, Fuxing Street, Guishan, Taoyuan 333, Taiwan; [c] Division of Sleep Medicine, Stanford University, 450 Broadway Pavillion C 2nd Floor, Redwood City, CA 94063, USA; [d] Department of Pediatric Dentistry, Chang Gung Memorial Hospital at Linkou, No. 5, Fuxing Street, Guishan, Taoyuan City 333, Taiwan; [e] Graduate Institute of Craniofacial and Dental Science, College of Medicine, Chang Gung University, 259 Wenhwa 1st Road, Guishan, Taoyuan 333, Taiwan

[1] Drs Huang and Hsu contributed equally to this work.

* Corresponding author. Department of Pediatric Dentistry, Chang Gung Memorial Hospital at Linkou, No. 5, Fuxing Street, Guishan, Taoyuan City 333, Taiwan.

E-mail address: soleus34@cgmh.org.tw

hypertrophy, obesity, anatomic and neuromuscular factors, and hypotonic neuromuscular diseases are also involved. Currently, the main cause of pediatric OSA is most commonly hypothesized to be a result of an anatomically or functionally narrowed upper airway. Related research in recent years showed that anatomic features of children with craniofacial anomalies are highly related to pediatric OSA.[9,10] Therefore, the established first-line treatment, adenotonsillectomy (AT), is unable to eradicate pediatric OSA completely, and high levels of relapse continue to be a point of contention.[11] There are very high rates of pediatric OSA in the preterm birth infant.[12] It means the initial oral facial anatomic build-up of an individual has a clear impact on the risk of collapsibility of the upper airway during sleep,[9,12] because there is a continuous interaction between orofacial functions and orofacial growth after birth. The dysfunctions identified to date affect orofacial development leading to SDB through changes in the orofacial growth.[9,10,12,13] Recently myofunctional therapy (MFT) has been suggested as an adjunct treatment of SDB in children.[9] Results of studies done on children with orthodontic problems have shown that isolated extensive and well-controlled MFT can lead to return to normal orofacial anatomy.[14] In adults, there is reported improvement of OSA and snoring also.[15–17] But the use of MFT alone when dealing with pediatric SDB has not been widely investigated and the long-term effects of MFT on SDB are still unknown. Problems with MFT have been reported: (1) current forms of MFT are difficult for children younger than 4 years, (2) the poor compliance with daily exercises and the absence of continuous parental involvement with the training exercises of the child are major causes of failure of treatment. Preliminary studies indicated that usage of a functional oral appliance thought to induce some extra muscle activity while asleep (also called "passive myofunctional therapy" [PMFT]) may decrease mouth breathing and have an impact on the position of the mandible.[16,17] Such changes may lead to improvement of the narrow upper-airway during sleep and may improve the snoring and pediatric OSA. The authors' study explored the effectiveness of MFT and PMFT on pediatric OSA and the long-term effects of these approaches on OSA and craniofacial growth.

METHODS

The study had the following design:

A. Patient recruitment
1. Children between 4 and 16 years of age, diagnosed with OSA based on clinical evaluation and nocturnal, in-laboratory polysomnography (PSG) with an apnea–hypopnea index (AHI) greater than 1 event/h or a respiratory disturbance index (RDI) greater than 5event/h; and
2. Either children previously diagnosed with pediatric OSA who had undergone adenotonsillectomy, but with residual AHI greater than 1 event/h or RDI greater than 5 event/h at 6 months after tonsillectomy and adenoidectomy (T&A) or children diagnosed with pediatric OSA but without evidence of adenotonsillar hypertrophy after ear, nose, and throat evaluation.
3. Recruited children were age matched and were treated (1) either with MFT (total 20 min/d) for 0.5 year (b) or with a previously described and specifically designed oral appliance with a tongue bead[18] during sleep (passive MFT) for 0.5 year. The appliance is a one-piece, custom-made adjustable oral device for advancing the mandible. A bead is mounted on the lower part of the frame for the tip of the tongue to roll, which in turn places the tongue in a forward position so as to open the airway.(c) The authors also recruited one age-match control group that did not receive any treatment and agreed to follow-up.
B. Procedures
Evaluation of the 3 groups was planned to be at baseline and subsequently at 3 and 6 months after MFT or PMFT treatment, with clinical evaluation, PSG, and lateral cephalometric films evaluating bone structure development at baseline, and 6 months.
C. PSG during sleep
A Neurovirtual BWIII PSG Plus sleep systemTM (Fort-Lauderdale. Fl. USA) was used. The following variables were recorded: electroencephalography (F3-M2, F4-M1, C3-M2, C4-M1, O1-M2, O2-M1), electro-oculogram (EOG), chin and leg electromyography (EMG), electrocardiography (ECG) with a modified V2 lead, body-position sensor, nasal cannula/pressure transducer, mouth thermistor, thoracic and abdominal plethysmography bands, neck microphone, and finger pulse oximetry.
Scoring was performed by an individual not involved in the study and blind to all conditions.
D. MFT
MFT is composed of isotonic and isometric exercises that target oral (lip, tongue) and oropharyngeal structures (soft palate,

lateral pharyngeal wall). MFT[14,17–19] aims to obtain appropriate head posture and positioning of the tongue on the palate against the upper teeth, appropriate swallowing and mastication using both sides and posterior chewing, appropriate breathing through the nose while keeping the mouth closed, and appropriate speech and articulation.

1. For soft palate exercises, patients pronounce oral vowel sounds either continuously (isometric exercises) or intermittently (isotonic exercises).[15]

2. Tongue exercises include moving the tongue along the superior and lateral surfaces of the teeth, positioning the tongue tip against the anterior aspect of the hard palate, pressing the entire tongue against the hard and soft palate, and forcing the tongue onto the floor of the mouth.[15]

3. Facial exercises address the lip (ie, contraction and relaxation of the orbicularis oris), buccinators (ie, suction movements and application of intraoral finger pressure against the buccinator muscles), and jaw muscles (ie, lateral jaw movements).[15]

4. Stomatognathic functions are addressed by instructing patients to inhale nasally and exhale orally without and then with balloon inflation and performing specific swallowing and chewing exercises (ie, swallowing with the teeth clenched together, tongue positioned in the palate, and without contraction of perioral muscles; alternating chewing sides).[15]

   For children, MFT requires active parental involvement to obtain good results. Parents and children had initial training with a specialist and parents were asked to supervise a minimum of 20 minutes of exercise daily. The MFT specialist was available to parents and regular clinical follow-up was scheduled. This regular daily activity was called "active MFT."[18]

E. Oral appliance

   The "passive MFT" short term used was reported recently.[18] The amount of mandibular advancement associated with the wearing of the device at rest-supine awake was 50% of the maximum mandibular advancement. Patients were instructed to wear their appliance nightly, the appliance been placed just at bedtime and to use their tongue to roll the bead (ie, passive MFT) just before falling asleep. Parents kept sleep logs to record

the nightly wear by all children for 12 months.

F. Statistical analysis

   General descriptive statistics, ANOVA, Wilcoxon signed-rank test, and Mann-Whitney analyses of the treatment results from the lateral cephalometric X ray, and PSG reports were performed using SPSS-18.

RESULTS

Total 121 pediatric OSA were enrolled. Fifty-four children were received MFT (Group A). But only 23 children completed the 6-month PSG study. Out of these 23, only 10 children had good compliance (compliance rate >80%) and completed pre- and postcephalometric test. Group B enrolled 56 pediatric OSA who received oral device (PMFT) treatment and 50 children completed 6 months of research with good compliance (>80%). The data showed no significant differences in age (groupA:7.02 ± 2.44; group B:7.97 ± 3.08, P = .338), sex (50% boy; 64.6% boy; P = .37), and BMI (16.61 ± 1.74; 17.82 ± 4.45, P = .10) distributions between the 2 groups. According to the questionnaires administered with oral device, children accepted nightly use of the device without complaint or objection. No side effect was reported by children or parents.

Considering the very important "drop-out" rate of subjects in Group A, the authors firstly performed analyses on Group A subjects. They considered each subject as its own control and compared baseline with posttreatment. PSG results are presented in **Table 1**. At 6-month follow-up, significant differences were already noted involving the respiratory disturbance index (P = .032), respiratory effort–related arousal (P = .048), and sleep latency (P = .036) that showed significant improvement after 0.5 year of treatment.

Interestingly the patients who received MFT and who had good compliance (n = 10) showed also significant improvement in AHI, PNS-NPhp (distance between PNS and posterior side of nasopharynx), and PNS-AD2 (distance from PNS to the nearest adenoid tissue measured along the line perpendicular to S-BA) measurements. Compared with no-treatment control group, the good compliance children in the Group A showed significant improvement in AHI (P = .037) (**Table 2**).

Table 3 shows the PSG outcome of 0.5 year of treatment with PMFT. Many significant findings were noted: significant decrease in the AHI during total sleep (P = .003), the hypopnea index (P = .003), the arousal index (P = .035), and the hypopnea count (P = .011).

Table 1
Polysomnography results of treatment with MFT

	PSG Pre (n = 23) Mean ± SD	PSG-0.5 y (n = 23) Mean ± SD	P-Value
BMI	16.61 ± 1.74	16.76 ± 2.12	.589
AHI in sleep (event/h)	2.47 ± 1.31	2.26 ± 1.84	.492
AHI in REM (event/h)	5.27 ± 4.15	4.99 ± 6.18	.799
AI (event/h)	1.43 ± 1.04	1.03 ± 02	.082
HI (event/h)	1.05 ± 0.92	1.23 ± 1.25	.518
ODI	1.64 ± 1.12	1.71 ± 2.22	.877
RDI	3.53 ± 2.01	2.57 ± 1.76	0.032*
Efficiency %	89.37 ± 5.01	90.41 ± 78.32	.312
Awake %	6.67 ± 4.58	7.04 ± 5.17	.759
REM %	24.31 ± 4.66	20.13 ± 7.0	.022*
Stage 1%	8.12 ± 4.43	12.15 ± 6.83	.041*
Stage 2%	38.82 ± 7.71	39.47 ± 9.87	.736
Stage 3%	28.75 ± 6.63	27.38 ± 7.53	.485
Total sleep time (min)	394.43 ± 22.73	398.33 ± 21.72	.504
Awake Count	12.70 ± 4.36	14.35 ± 5.52	.170
Sleep Latency (min)	16.20 ± 12.83	10.78 ± 9.49	.036*
REM Latency (min)	64.5 ± 27.16	94.5 ± 56.34	.023*
Arousal Count	43.83 ± 14.27	40.52 ± 11.15	.321
Arousal Index	7.96 ± 2.74	7.2 ± 1.97	.219
Mean Heart Rate	82.14 ± 14.04	78.23 ± 10.67	.098
PLM Index (event/h)	0.30 ± 1.00	1.14 ± 2.66	.124
Snore Index (event/h)	136.32 ± 144.80	122.38 ± 123.58	.683
Obstructive Apnea	0.39 ± 0.78	0.48 ± 0.99	.648
Central Apnea	6.87 ± 5.50	4.91 ± 5.53	.161
Mixed Apnea	0.74 ± 1.86	0.48 ± 0.85	.503
Hypopnea	5.87 ± 5.11	6.91 ± 7.17	.515
RERA	5.87 ± 8.96	1.74 ± 2.78	.048*
Mean SaO2%	97.74 ± 0.62	97.83 ± 0.39	.539

t-test was performed to analyze the 0.5 year of treatment results.
Abbreviations: AI, apnea index; HI, hypopnea index; mean SaO2, mean oxygen saturation; ODI, oxygen desaturation index; PLMS index, periodic leg movements in sleep index; RDI, respiratory disturbance index; REM, rapid eye movement; RERA, respiratory effort–related arousal.
* $P<.05$.

The authors could compare only the children with good compliances for MFT (ie, n = 10) and the subjects who used the device regularly (ie, n = 48). It is obvious that the improvement of AHI and upper airway of group B (passive MFT) is more than group A (MFT) (see **Tables 1** and **3**).

DISCUSSION

In adults, there is reported improvement of OSA and snoring under MFT, but MFT alone when dealing with pediatric SDB has not been widely investigated.[15–17] Moreover, the long-term effect

on SDB is unknown. Prior publications looking at role of MFT in improving sleep-related breathing had emphasized the very large amount of nonusable data.[15,17,19–21] Compliance with treatment is a major issue. In prior studies the authors learned that it is very important, particularly at the beginning of treatment, to see child and parents several times a week and to involve in depth one of the parents who will perform the exercise at the same time as the child. Such involvement may be costly depending of the social security system and the reimbursement provided for the specialist involvement. The daily involvement of at least one parent with performance of the

Table 2
Comparison of the difference of cephalometric outcome between the treatment with myofunctional therapy (good compliance) and control group

	MFT (Good Compliance) (n = 10)			Control (n = 11)			MFT 0.5y-Pre Mean ± SD	Control 0.5y-Pre Mean ± SD	P_T Value
	Ceph-Pre Mean ± SD	Ceph-0.5 y Mean ± SD	P Value	Ceph-Pre Mean ± SD	Ceph-0.5 y Mean ± SD	P Value			
Age	6.8 ± 1.99	—	—	8.46 ± 3.00	—	—	—	—	0.443
Gender (Male %)	40.0%	—	—	72.7%	—	—	—	—	0.096
AHI (event/h)	2.46 ± 1.52	1.46 ± 1.41	.015*	2.42 ± 2.83	2.59 ± 2.11	.766	−1.00 ± 1.18	0.17 ± 2.09	0.037*
AI	1.11 ± 0.94	0.60 ± 0.61	.249	0.76 ± 0.78	0.93 ± 0.55	.483	−0.51 ± 1.08	0.23 ± 0.94	0.246
ODI	1.60 ± 1.04	1.04 ± 1.49	.208	2.13 ± 3.07	2.04 ± 2.37	.859	−0.56 ± 1.82	0.23 ± 3.00	0.248
HI	0.78 ± 0.54	0.49 ± 0.45	.058	2.32 ± 3.03	1.40 ± 1.96	.483	0.29 ± 0.46	−0.83 ± 3.21	0.595
ANB	6.67 ± 2.16	6.60 ± 2.02	.779	4.92 ± 2.19	4.78 ± 2.46	.441	−0.07 ± 0.82	−0.14 ± 1.37	0.620
PNS-NPhp	11.64 ± 3.81	13.66 ± 3.81	.028*	12.55 ± 4.12	14.26 ± 4.16	.131	2.02 ± 2.45	1.70 ± 4.40	0.526
PMm-NPh	6.40 ± 3.30	7.55 ± 3.00	.103	9.75 ± 2.90	9.78 ± 3.76	.859	1.15 ± 1.82	0.02 ± 2.88	0.439
OPha-OPhp	11.87 ± 5.67	9.63 ± 2.07	.241	13.44 ± 3.96	11.18 ± 1.71	.041*	−2.25 ± 5.51	−2.26 ± 3.17	0.647
MinRGA	12.87 ± 3.33	11.99 ± 2.20	.508	14.31 ± 3.49	12.72 ± 2.78	.213	−0.88 ± 3.25	−1.59 ± 3.35	0.673
PNS-AD2	11.15 ± 2.58	13.23 ± 2.99	.028*	12.82 ± 3.97	14.12 ± 3.07	.026*	2.09 ± 2.23	1.30 ± 1.47	0.324

Abbreviations: AI, apnea index; ANB, A point-nasion-B point angle (normal range is about 2–4); HI, hypopnea index; MinRGA, minimal retroglossal airway; ODI, oxygen desaturation index; OPha-OPhp, distance anterior side-posterior side of oropharynx; P, Intragroup comparison: Wilcoxon signed-rank test; PMm-NPh, distance soft palate-posterior side of nasopharynx; PNS-AD2, distance from PNS to the nearest adenoid tissue measured along the line perpendicular to S-BA; PNS- NPhp, distance between PNS and posterior side of nasopharynx; P_T, intergroup comparison: Mann-Whitney test for difference between groups.
  * P<.05.

Table 3
Polysomnography results of treatment with oral device (passive myofunctional therapy)

	PSG Pre(n = 50) Mean ± SD	PSG 0.5 y(n = 50) Mean ± SD	P-Value
BMI	17.82 ± 4.45	18.26 ± .50	.124
AHI in sleep	5.56 ± 6.65	2.85 ± 2.45	.003**
AHI in REM	9.64 ± 12.32	7.59 ± 9.29	.126
AI	1.47 ± 2.25	1.01 ± 1.12	.131
HI	3.46 ± 4.45	1.84 ± 1.95	.003**
ODI	4.03 ± 6.72	2.71 ± 3.17	.133
RDI	7.41 ± 10.85	5.34 ± 4.11	.237
Efficiency %	86.01 ± 11.44	87.85 ± 9.77	.328
Awake %	10.57 ± 11.11	7.89 ± 7.06	.130
REM %	20.44 ± 4.99	19.35 ± 5.29	.054
Stage 1%	9.29 ± 7.38	9.47 ± 6.52	.867
Stage 2%	43.36 ± 8.91	44.87 ± 8.40	.336
Stage 3%	25.89 ± 9.14	26.29 ± 8.04	.780
Total Sleep Time	389.37 ± 59.76	390.16 ± 60.73	.947
Awake Count	17.67 ± 10.13	17.71 ± 11.41	.984
Sleep Latency	14.08 ± 12.07	17.44 ± 20.30	.312
REM Latency	108.49 ± 74.83	95.74 ± 57.51	.280
Arousal Index	11.02 ± 8.50	9.02 ± 5.17	.035*
Mean Heart Rate	74.24 ± 13.19	69.94 ± 14.81	.058
PLM Index	0.99 ± 2.74	0.56 ± 1.58	.267
Snore Index	142.65 ± 205.37	123.78 ± 155.01	.477
Obstructive Apnea	3.02 ± 7.83	1.42 ± 3.68	.127
Central Apnea	4.20 ± 6.01	4.02 ± 4.85	.841
Mixed Apnea	1.34 ± 3.93	0.50 ± 1.18	.166
Hypopnea	17.96 ± 23.14	10.54 ± 11.18	.011*
RERA	17.79 ± 20.74	15.33 ± 18.95	.464
Mean SaO2%	97.38 ± 0.67	96.93 ± 4.24	.467
WASO	32.36 ± 4.76	28.93 ± 28.19	.631

PSG-0.5 y: PSG was performed with usage of oral device at the time of recording.
ANOVA. Post hoc: Bonferroni test.
Abbreviations: AI, apnea index; HI, hypopnea index; Mean SaO2, mean oxygen saturation; ODI, oxygen desaturation index; PLMS index, periodic leg movements in sleep index; RDI, respiratory disturbance index; RERA, respiratory effort–related arousal.
* $P<.05$.
** $P<.01$.

exercises at the same time in the morning and/or evening with the child is a critical issue. Social factors are important in MFT—often both parents work outside; families may have several children; work and school schedules—but, particularly in Far East Asian countries, the very large demands from schools and very demanding home-work time are clear handicap to parental involvement in daily reeducation programs. Even in the 10 families where good compliance was noted at 6 months, the authors were unable to pursue their long-term follow-up. MFT is one of the rehabilitations, and there is no way to get the immediate results; therefore many parents or patients easily give up after 3 months of treatment. The "passive MFT" requires very little involvement of parents, and children are very quickly used of having the device in their mouth, so compliance is not a problem. But placing any dental device in a mouth of a child is always an issue: any effect induced on one of the jaw will lead quickly to a compensatory effect on the other one. Many devices are advertised for children, but very little, if any, study has been performed to appreciate the long-term changes induces on upper and lower jaws when an appliance is used for several months, despite the fact that such changes are always noted to some degree after months of usage. The authors kept their device for 0.5 year and could not see any change at their clinical and imaging evaluations. But they used cephalometric X rays and probably in the future 3-dimensional dental computed tomography will be a better tool. Usage of such devices must be done with clear follow-up and usage must be with clear time limit. Also long-term follow-up without any of these devices is an important issue.

How the device really works has not been completely worked out. It is a type of "functional appliance," and functional appliances have been "advertised" for more than 70 years,[22] as having effects on orofacial growth, but the secondary effects noted when usage is too long and the unavoidable impact on the other jaw has been clear limitation in their usage.

One crucial finding with the PSG at 0.5 year postrecording compared with baseline is that they breathed through their nose during sleep, while mouth breathing was the rule at baseline including in our post-T&A children. All-night nasal breathing is the only demonstration of successful treatment of the upper airway.[23]

Finally, the authors' study is the first prospective study performed on children with pediatric OSA that demonstrate that MFT can lead to nasal breathing during sleep. It also outlined the very important difficulties associated with such treatment. The limitations are the high drop-out rate of MFT group and the authors only followed 6 months side effect of oral device treatment (PMFT). This study indicates that "passive MFT" may be a valid alternative, but very careful attention to the potential negative secondary impact of the device, that may not be immediately appreciated, is a clear requirement.

ACKNOWLEDGMENTS

These data were presented at the "The International Pediatric Sleep Association", Paris, April, 2018.

REFERENCES

1. Young T, Palta M, Dempsey J, et al. The occurrence of sleep-disordered breathing among middle-aged adults. N Engl J Med 1993;328:1230–5.

2. Dempsey JA, Veasey SC, Morgan BJ, et al. Pathophysiology of sleep apnea. Physiol Rev 2010;90: 47–112.

3. Sullivan CE, Issa FG, Berthon-Jones M, et al. Reversal of obstructive sleep apnoea by continuous positive airway pressure applied through the nares. Lancet 1981;1:862–5.

4. Camacho M, Certal V, Capasso R. Comprehensive review of surgeries for obstructive sleep apnea syndrome. Braz J Otorhinolaryngol 2013;79: 780–8.

5. Randerath WJ, Verbraecken J, Andreas S, et al. Non-CPAP therapies in obstructive sleep apnoea. Eur Respir J 2011;37:1000–28.

6. Guilleminault C, Eldridge FL, Simmons FB, et al. Sleep apnea in eight children. Pediatrics 1976;58: 23–30.

7. Guilleminault C, Lee JH, Chan A. Pediatric obstructive sleep apnea syndrome. Arch Pediatr Adolesc Med 2005;159:775–85.

8. Marcus CL, Brooks LJ, Draper KA, et al. Clinical practice guideline. Diagnosis and management of childhood obstructive sleep apnea syndrome. Pediatrics 2012;130:576–84.

9. Guilleminault C, Huang YS. From oral facial dysfunction to dysmorphism and the onset of pediatric OSA. Sleep Med Rev 2018;40:203–14.

10. Huang YS, Guilleminault C. Pediatric obstructive sleep apnea and the critical role of oralfacial growth: evidences. Front Neurol 2012;3:184.

11. Huang YS, Guilleminault C, Lee LA, et al. Treatment outcomes of adenotonsillectomy for children with obstructive sleep apnea: a prospective longitudinal study. Sleep 2014;37:71–6.

12. Huang YS, Paiva T, Hsu TF, et al. Sleep and breathing in premature infants at 6 months post-natal age. BMC Pediatr 2014;14:303–9.

13. Jamieson A, Guilleminault C, Partinen M, et al. Obstructive sleep apneic patients have craniomandibular abnormalities. Sleep 1986;9:469–77.

14. Chauvois A, Fournier M, Girardin F. Reeducation des fonctionsdans la therapeutique orthodontiques. Paris: S.I.D; 1999.

15. Guimarães KC, Drager LF, Genta PR, et al. Effects of oropharyngeal exercises on patients with moderate obstructive sleep apnea syndrome. Am J Respir Crit Care Med 2009;179:962–6.

16. Guilleminault C, Akhtar F. Pediatrics sleep-disordered-breathing: new evidences on its development. Sleep Med Rev 2015;14:1–11.

17. Villa MP, Evangelisti M, Martella S, et al. Can myofunctional therapy increase tongue tone and reduce symptoms in children with sleep-disordered breathing? Sleep Breath 2017;21(4): 1025–32.

18. Chuang LC, Lian YC, Hervy-Auboiron M, et al. Passive myofunctional therapy applied on children with

obstructive sleep apnea: a 6-month follow-up. J Formos Med Assoc 2017;116:536–41.

19. Camacho M, Certal V, Abdullatif J, et al. Myofunctional therapy to treat obstructive sleep apnea: a systematic review and meta-analysis. Sleep 2015; 38:669–75.

20. Guilleminault C, Huang YS, Quo S, et al. Teenage sleep disordered breathing: recurrence of syndrome. Sleep Med 2013;14:37–44.

21. Guilleminault C, Huang YS, Monteyrol PJ, et al. Critical role of myofacial reeducation in sleep-disordered breathing. Sleep Med 2013;14: 518–25.

22. Schwartz M, Acosta L, Hung YL, et al. Effects of CPAP and mandibular advancement device treatment in obstructive sleep apnea patients: a systematic review and meta-analysis Sleep. Breath 2018; 22(3):555–68.

23. Sullivan SS, Guilleminault C. Can we avoid development of a narrow upper airway and secondary abnormal breathing during sleep? Lancet Respir Med 2017;5:843–4.

Weight Management in Obstructive Sleep Apnea
Medical and Surgical Options

Kwang Wei Tham, MB, BCh, BAO, ABIM*,
Phong Ching Lee, MBChB, FRCP (Edin),
Chin Hong Lim, MB, Bh, BAO, FRCA

KEYWORDS

- Obesity • Weight loss • Obstructive sleep apnea • Bariatric surgery • Pharmacotherapy • Asians

KEY POINTS

- Obesity plays a pivotal role in the pathogenesis of obstructive sleep apnea (OSA) and weight loss of approximately 7% to 11% leads to clinically significant and meaningful improvement in OSA.
- Lifestyle modification with reduced calorie intake and increased physical activity forms the foundation of all weight loss interventions and seems to have weight-independent benefits in OSA.
- Pharmacotherapy for obesity management alters energy regulation usually by reducing appetite and increasing satiety and should be considered an adjunct to lifestyle intervention.
- Bariatric surgery provides the largest amount of weight loss and should be considered in clinically severe obesity (body mass index $\geq$35 kg/m^2 or $\geq$32.5 kg/m^2 in Asians) with OSA or other obesity-related complications.
- A patient-centric approach with goals meaningful to patients, such as improvement of OSA and improvement in quality of life, should be the guiding principle in obesity management in OSA.

INTRODUCTION

In 2016, the World Health Organization estimated that the global prevalence of overweight and obesity had reached 39% and 13%, respectively, with 52% either overweight or obese.[1] With drastic changes in the environment, food industry, and dietary and physical activity patterns, the worldwide obesity prevalence has nearly tripled since 1975.[1] Based on Organisation for Economic Co-operation and Development estimates in 2015, the United States, New Zealand, Hungary, and Mexico have attained obesity rates of more than 30% whereas Asian countries like China, Japan, and Korea have a lower prevalence of less than 7%.[2] Global obesity rates are projected to rise

further, with the largest risk in developing rural areas and in children, posing potential threats to greater noncommunicable disease burden and health care costs.[1]

In tandem with the rise in obesity, the prevalence of obesity-related diseases, such as obstructive sleep apnea (OSA), has synchronously increased. Excess adiposity has undoubtedly been established as the most crucial causal factor of OSA and 60% to 70% of individuals with OSA are overweight or obese.[3–5] In 1993, the estimated prevalence of sleep-disordered breathing (SDB) (defined as an apnea-hypopnea index [AHI] of $\geq$5/h) was 9% in women and 24% in men in the Wisconsin Sleep Cohort.[6] Approximately 20 years on, the estimated prevalence has risen to 17% and

Disclosure Statement: Dr K.W. Tham has served on the advisory board or as a speaker of Novo Nordisk (Singapore), Johnson & Johnson, Merck Sharp & Dohme, and Sanofi.
The Academia, 20 College Road, Singapore 169856, Singapore
* Corresponding author.
E-mail address: tham.kwang.wei@singhealth.com.sg

Sleep Med Clin 14 (2019) 143–153
https://doi.org/10.1016/j.jsmc.2018.10.002
1556-407X/19/© 2018 Elsevier Inc. All rights reserved.

34% in women and men, respectively.[7] A similarly large increase in incidence of OSA in Asia is expected, given the recent, rapid rise in obesity rates throughout Asia.[8]

With obesity the most modifiable risk factor of OSA, the treatment of obesity with weight loss is fundamental in the management of a majority of patients with OSA. This article aims to discuss the relationship of obesity and OSA, the various interventions currently available in the treatment of obesity, and the approach to obesity management in OSA.

IMPACT OF OBESITY ON OBSTRUCTIVE SLEEP APNEA

Impact on Prevalence of Obstructive Sleep Apnea, Its Severity, and Its Progression

It is well recognized that obesity is a seminal factor in the pathogenesis of OSA and reported to be the most important predictor of SDB in population studies.[9] Approximately 58% of moderate to severe OSA cases are attributable to excess adiposity and weight.[5] The degree of obesity augments the severity of OSA. The prevalence of OSA in the general population is estimated at 15%. Among obese adult cohorts, the prevalence is doubled to 30%. In patients with clinically severe obesity, particularly those presenting for bariatric surgery, the prevalence is even higher, at 60% to 86%.[9–11]

In the Wisconsin Sleep Cohort, the prevalence of SDB is more than doubled in men with body mass index (BMI) 30 kg/m^2 to 39.9 kg/m^2 (class I and II obesity) compared with overweight men (BMI 25–29.9 kg/m^2), from 18.3% to 44.6%.[7] Weight gain over time is also predictive of OSA development; in an earlier study of the same cohort, a 10% increase in body weight was associated with a 6-fold increase in the risk of developing sleep apnea over a 4-year period, and a rise in AHI by 32%.[6]

Adding Weight to the Pathophysiology

The pathogenesis of OSA is complex and involves a dynamic interplay of anatomic, mechanical, functional (neuromuscular), and dynamic airway abnormalities.

Increase in body adiposity leads to deposition of fatty tissue within the airway and pharyngeal walls with consequential reduction in luminal diameter of the pharynx. There is an increase in upper airway collapsibility from a reduced upper airway muscle protective force and even structural and functional anomalies in the dilator muscles of the pharynx, which may additionally be related to an increase in orexin effect. Systemic and local inflammatory factors as a result of obesity may exacerbate these factors. Accumulation of abdominal fat, especially visceral fat, results in mass effect on the chest wall and a reduced functional residual volume.[9,12]

OSA as Metabolic Partners in Crime

Obesity is central to the pathogenesis of a constellation of conditions, such as insulin resistance, type 2 diabetes mellitus (T2DM), dyslipidemia, hypertension (HTN), and nonalcoholic fatty liver disease (NAFLD). These individually and compositely lead to an increased risk of cardiovascular disease (CVD) and mortality.[13,14]

OSA finds itself in association with these CV risk factors through its common root of obesity and by itself is a risk factor for various types of CVD. Presence of morbid obesity aggravates OSA and fuels the associated conditions of insulin resistance, T2DM, dyslipidemia, and HTN, spiraling the untreated patient down a vicious cycle with a compounded risk of end-organ diseases like renal impairment, heart failure, stroke, and ischemic heart disease.[14]

IMPACT OF OBSTRUCTIVE SLEEP APNEA ON OBESITY

Often neglected is the potential reciprocal impact of OSA on obesity, suggesting the relationship between obesity and OSA may well be synergistic.[15]

OSA predisposes individuals to the development and worsening of obesity. Consequential to intermittent hypoxia, sleep deprivation and fragmentation, and disrupted metabolism in OSA, associated changes in cortisol, leptin, orexin, and ghrelin levels, with subsequent increase in hunger and caloric intake, have been reported.[16] Other studies have noted a higher energy intake and preference for caloric-dense food, with a higher incidence of disinhibited eating behavior, hence an increase in the risk of or aggravation of obesity.[9,15,17,18]

PRINCIPLES OF WEIGHT LOSS IN OBSTRUCTIVE SLEEP APNEA

Given the important link between obesity and OSA, weight loss is the most logical clinical recommendation for overweight and obese patients with OSA.

Weight loss benefits OSA and significantly improves the concomitant obesity-related conditions. Hence, weight loss is multipurpose and sets the patient into a healthier cycle with the ultimate goal of improving health and quality of life and reducing end-organ sequelae.[19,20]

The aim of weight loss should always be set clearly with a patient when deciding the optimal weight loss approach. There has been a recent shift in treatment paradigm, adopting a patient-centric rather than a BMI-centric approach (which focuses on a predetermined amount of weight loss). Prevention of disease progression and complications and amelioration of the obesity-related disease hence become the main goals of weight loss interventions.[20]

IMPACT OF WEIGHT LOSS ON OBSTRUCTIVE SLEEP APNEA

Weight loss of 5% to 10% leads to improvement in obesity-related medical conditions in many patients, including OSA, T2DM, insulin resistance, and HTN.[21–23] For clinically significant and meaningful improvement in OSA, the weight loss goal should be at least 7% to 11%.[20]

Regardless of type of weight loss intervention, the greatest benefits are in those who achieve greater weight loss and those with more severe OSA. Remission of OSA is achievable, more likely in those who lose more weight and with initial mild OSA.[24,25] One year after bariatric surgery, subjects lost a mean of 25% of their weight and 45% of patients experienced OSA remission. Beyond 27% weight loss, there was no further increase in AHI reduction, suggesting that the maximal benefit of weight loss on AHI improvement may be capped at approximately 25 to 30% weight loss.[26]

Each weight loss intervention produces variable results in each individual. It is pertinent to assess the status of the patient—severity of OSA and coexistence of other obesity-related diseases—to decide on the most appropriate therapy for the best result in that patient.

WEIGHT LOSS INTERVENTIONS IN OBSTRUCTIVE SLEEP APNEA
Lifestyle Interventions: The Importance of Diet and Exercise

Lifestyle modification with reduced calorie intake and increased physical activity forms the foundation of all weight loss interventions on which adjunctive therapy, like pharmacotherapy and/or bariatric surgery, is built.[2]

Several observational studies and randomized controlled trials (RCTs) have studied the effect of lifestyle intervention and weight loss on OSA.[27] In the Sleep AHEAD (Action for Health in Diabetes) RCT, a multicenter ancillary investigation of the Look AHEAD trial, 264 overweight/obese patients with T2DM and OSA were randomized to receive either diabetes support and education or intensive lifestyle intervention (ILI).[11] The ILI consisted of a reduced-calorie diet of 1200 kcal per day to 1800 kcal per day with the use of meal replacements and at least 175 minutes of moderate-intensity physical activity per week.[23] At 1 year, the ILI group, which achieved an average weight loss of 10.5%, was more than 3 times more likely to achieve total remission of their OSA and had AHI that was 9.7 events/h lower than the diabetes support and education group (P<.001). Initial AHI and weight loss were the strongest predictors of changes in AHI at 1 year, and those who achieved weight loss of 10 kg or more had the greatest reductions in AHI.[11] There seems to be a linear relationship between weight loss and change in AHI across the spectrum of OSA severity, with AHI reduction of approximately 0.4 events/h/kg weight loss.[11,28]

These benefits were subsequently maintained over a 4-year period, despite an almost 50% weight regain. Remission of OSA was 5 times more likely in the ILI subjects (20.7%) compared with controls (3.6%).[25] Beneficial effects from improved fitness, increase physical activity, and adherence to prescribed advice are possible reasons for this sustained effect other than weight loss. Hence, it is important to adopt a structured, holistic approach in addition to weight reduction in management of patients with OSA.

Specific Dietary Interventions and Obstructive Sleep Apnea

The conventional hypocaloric diet of 1200 kcal to 1800 kcal daily leads to modest weight loss and has been studied in numerous weight loss trials, including Look AHEAD and the Diabetes Prevention Program. Many other popular diets (with different macronutrient compositions), however, exist. A meta-analysis has shown that significant weight loss was observed with any low-carbohydrate or low-fat diet and that the best diet for any given patient is a diet that a person can adhere to.[29] Nevertheless, the specific dietary interventions discussed in this article have been studied in relation to OSA.

Very-low-calorie diet
The nonsurgical interventions that produce the most dramatic weight loss over a short-term period of 6 months involve the use of very-low-calorie diets (VLCDs), which provide fewer than 800 kcal/d.[30] This medically supervised diet is achieved using specially formulated and nutritionally complete meal replacements. Since the 1970s, VLCDs have been used to induce safe and rapid weight loss, while preserving lean body mass.[31]

The rapid weight loss that can be achieved with VLCD also does not seem to affect the rate of weight regain compared with a conventional gradual weight loss program.[32] VLCD-induced weight loss significantly improved OSA and other measures of autonomic nervous system, such as blood pressure and baroreflex sensitivity.[33] In moderate to severe OSA, a structured VLCD program led to 17% weight loss with an associated 67% reduction in AHI in just 9 weeks,[24] with sustained benefits even after 1 year.[34]

Mediterranean diet

The traditional Mediterranean diet is characterized by a high intake of olive oil, fruit, nuts, vegetables, and grains; a moderate intake of fish and poultry; a low intake of dairy products, red meat, processed meats, and sweets; and moderate intake of wine taken together with meals.[35] The diet has several purported health benefits, including reduction in the incidence of cardiovascular events in those at high cardiovascular risk[36] and prevention of T2DM[37] as well as improvement in metabolic syndrome[38] and NAFLD.[39]

The benefits of Mediterranean diet also seem to extend to OSA, with greater improvement in AHI during rapid eye movement sleep at 6 months.[40] It has been postulated that these benefits may be independent of weight loss and potential mechanisms involve redistribution of body fat and reductions in oxidative stress, and inflammation, leading to improvement in upper airway neuromuscular control and upper airway muscle force-generating capacity.[41]

Physical Activity: Improvement in Obstructive Sleep Apnea Beyond Weight Loss

Guidelines recommend moderate-intensity physical activity of at least 150 minutes a week or vigorous-intensity physical activity for at least 60 minutes a week as part of a healthy lifestyle.[42] Although exercise does not usually lead to significant changes in body weight, there is robust evidence that regular physical activity plays an important role in the primary and secondary prevention of chronic diseases, such as CVD, diabetes, cancer, HTN, obesity, depression, and osteoporosis.[43] Similarly, there seem to be weight-independent effects of physical activity on improvements in several parameters of OSA,[44] including AHI and oxygen saturation.[45] Several mechanisms have been proposed; these include improvement in muscle tone of the upper airways,[46,47] reduction in nocturnal rostral fluid shift,[48] and a profound effect on central adiposity.[41]

Effect of Obstructive Sleep Apnea as Moderator of Lifestyle-Induced Weight Loss

Although it is clear that lifestyle intervention via diet and physical activity improves OSA, the relationship also seems bidirectional, with attenuation of diet-induced weight loss in patients with OSA.[41] In men with visceral obesity, OSA attenuates improvements in lipid profile and glucose levels.[49] These findings could potentially be explained by the effects of changes in energy expenditure,[15] in disrupted sleep on appetite hormones,[16] and on sympathetic nervous activity, leading to increased cortisol levels and insulin resistance.[50]

Given the deleterious effects of OSA on weight loss efforts, it is plausible to consider adding continuous positive airway pressure (CPAP) therapy in the management of obesity. The results thus far, however, have been mixed. RCTs have shown that CPAP alone without diet or exercise,[51] or used in conjunction with cognitive behavioral therapy, does not lead to weight loss.[52] When used in conjunction with a weight-loss program, however, CPAP provided an incremental reduction in insulin resistance, serum triglyceride levels, and blood pressure compared with either intervention alone.[53]

Pharmacotherapy

Although lifestyle intervention remains the foundation of obesity management, following an exemplary diet and exercise recommendations produces only modest weight loss that is difficult to sustain in a majority of patients. This is due to the multitude of physiologic neurohormonal changes in response to weight loss that increase energy intake and reduce energy expenditure.[54,55] Hence, additional therapeutic approaches beyond lifestyle interventions are often required to produce clinically significant weight loss.

Pharmacotherapy for obesity management should be used as an adjunct to lifestyle intervention just as it is for managing other chronic diseases, such as HTN, diabetes, and CVD, and not as a substitute treatment modality. Weight loss medications alter energy regulation usually by reducing appetite, allowing satiation with a smaller meal and more prolonged satiety after a small meal. These pharmacologic agents produce approximately 5% to 15% weight loss over 1 year when used in conjunction with lifestyle intervention.[56]

Weight loss pharmacotherapy should be considered for individuals with BMI greater than 30 kg/m^2 or with BMI greater than 27 kg/m^2 with obesity-related complications.[22,57,58] In Asian populations, the BMI thresholds should be lowered to BMI greater than 27 kg/m^2 or BMI greater than 25 kg/m^2 with complications. Currently, 5 types of medications are approved by the US Food and Drug Administration for long-term treatment of obesity and include lipase inhibitors (orlistat), a combination of phentermine–topiramate, glucagon-like peptide 1 (GLP-1) receptor agonists (liraglutide at 3 mg/d dose), serotonin 2C receptor agonists (lorcaserin), and combination of naltrexone–bupropion.[57] The dosages, average weight loss, common side effects, and contraindications for these medications are shown in **Table 1**. Choice of pharmacotherapy should be tailored to patient needs, taking into consideration patient baseline profile and coexisting medical problems to ensure the best efficacy and least adverse effects for patients.

An RCT involving moderate to severe OSA patients has shown improvement in OSA and related symptoms with the phentermine–topiramate combination compared with placebo, and the effects were mediated by weight loss.[59] Similarly, the SCALE Sleep Apnea RCT showed that liraglutide produced significantly greater reductions than placebo in AHI and body weight in patients with obesity and moderate/severe OSA.[60] Beyond weight loss, liraglutide also has glucose-lowering and cardiovascular benefits, including reduction in CV mortality and CVD events in patients with T2DM.[61,62]

Patients should be reviewed closely for the first 3 months on commencement of pharmacotherapy to assess safety, tolerability, and efficacy. The medication should be stopped immediately should any safety or significant tolerability issues arise. There is also significant variability in individual weight-loss responses to these medications. It has been shown that weight loss at 12 weeks to 16 weeks predicts later weight loss at 1 year and beyond.[63] Therefore, if a patient's response is insufficient (weight loss <5% at 3–4 months) despite optimization of adherence and dose, the medication should be stopped because the long-term risks and costs of therapy likely outweigh the benefits. On the other hand, if the treatment is shown effective and well-tolerated, it should be continued. This is akin to diabetes and HTN management, whereby antihyperglycemic and antihypertensive medications are continued even after glycemic or blood pressure targets have been attained.

Bariatric Surgery: Last but Not the Least

Currently, the 2 most commonly performed bariatric procedures are sleeve gastrectomy (SG) and Roux-en-Y gastric bypass (RYGB). Surgical alteration of the anatomy of the gastrointestinal tract affects the body's absorption and handling of nutrients as well as powerful neurohormonal changes that influence hunger and satiety, leading to weight loss (**Fig. 1**).

SG restricts the volume capacity of the stomach to just 100 mL (previously approximately 2000 mL), resulting in early satiety, therefore reducing caloric consumption.[64] RYGB exerts its effects via a combination of volume restriction and by bypassing 150 cm to 200 cm of small intestine.[65]

Bariatric surgery primarily works by restricting caloric intake and via changes in key hormones that occur after surgical manipulation of the gut, which are related to energy balance and weight loss. Changes in these hormones after the common surgical procedures are shown in **Table 2**.

Expected weight loss after bariatric surgery

Most of the weight loss occurs in the first 2 years after surgery. In fact, 60% of excess weight loss (excess weight = preoperative weight – weight at ideal BMI) occurs in the first 6 months after surgery and 77% occurs as early as the first 12 months.[66] Patients maintain on average at least 50% excess weight loss 5 years postoperative. This is seen in both SG and RYGB surgery. The Swedish Obese Subjects study, the longest prospective case-control study of various types of bariatric surgery, reported an average weight loss of 32% 15 years after RYGB.[67] In the Asian population, higher weight loss was observed in RYGB compared with SG after 3 years, and this continued up to 5 years postoperatively.[68]

Metabolic surgery: the strength of bariatric surgery and its impact on obstructive sleep apnea

After bariatric surgery, improvements in metabolic conditions, including T2DM, dyslipidemia, OSA, and NAFLD, has been tremendous such that resolution of these conditions is often seen. This has led to bariatric surgery being recommended as a therapeutic option and renamed metabolic surgery.[66–68]

In a study comparing gastric bypass versus ILI for OSA, bariatric surgery provided better weight loss than ILI (30% vs 8%) and greater remission of OSA of 66% versus 40% in ILI. This suggests that perhaps moderate weight loss in OSA is sufficient to improve OSA severity and that greater weight loss beyond 25% to 30% does not confer better benefit.[69]

The impact of different bariatric procedures on OSA seems to be differing. A systemic review

Table 1
Pharmacotherapy for obesity approved for chronic use in the United States

Drug	Dose	Weight Loss vs Placebo	Side Effects	Contraindications
Orlistat	120 mg TDS	2.9%–3.4% at 1 y	Steatorrhea, oily spotting, flatulence with discharge, fecal incontinence, fat-soluble vitamin malabsorption	Pregnancy
Phe/Top	Phe 3.75 mg/top 23 mg OD (starting dose) Phe 7.5 mg/top 46 mg OD (recommended dose) Phe 15 mg/top 92 mg mane (high dose)	5.0%–6.6% at 1 y	Phe: dry mouth, insomnia, agitation, constipation, and tachycardia Top: paraesthesia, dry mouth, constipation, altered taste sensation, insomnia, dizziness, cognitive effects Rare: closed angle glaucoma, depression/suicidal ideation	Phe: severe HTN, CVD, glaucoma, history of drug/alcohol abuse, MAO inhibitors, SSRI use, pregnancy Top: glaucoma, renal stones, pregnancy (if used for weight loss)
Liraglutide	Up-titrate gradually to 3.0 mg OD	5.4% at 1 y	Nausea, vomiting, diarrhea, constipation Rare: pancreatitis, cholecystitis	Severe renal or hepatic insufficiency, pregnancy, past history of pancreatitis and major depression or psychiatric disorder
Lorcaserin	12.5 mg BD	3.6% at 1 y	Headache, nausea, dry mouth, dizziness, fatigue, constipation	Pregnancy Use with caution: other serotonergic or antidopaminergic agents, St John's wort, triptans, bupropion, dextromethorphan
Naltrexone/bupropion	32 mg/360 mg 2 tablets OD (high dose)	4.8% at 1 y	Nausea, constipation, headache, vomiting, dizziness Rare: suicidal thoughts/behaviours	Uncontrolled HTN, seizure disorders, anorexia nervosa or bulimia, chronic opioid use, MAO inhibitors

Abbreviations: BD, twice daily; CVD, cardiovascular disease; HTN, hypertension; MAO, monoamine oxidase; OD, once daily; Phe, phentermine; SSRI, selective serotonin reuptake inhibitor; TDS, three times a day; Top, topiramate.
From Papandreou C, Schiza SE, Bouloukaki I, et al. Effect of Mediterranean diet versus prudent diet combined with physical activity on OSAS: a randomised trial. Eur Respir J 2012;39(6):1398–404; with permission. Reproduced with permission of the © ERS 2018: European Respiratory Journal Jun 2012;39(6):1398–404; DOI: 10.1183/09031936.00103411.

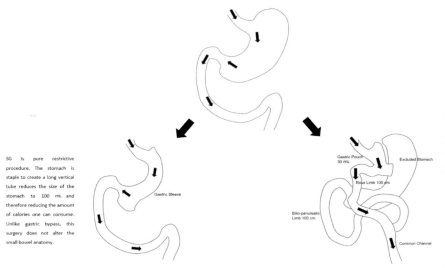

SG is pure restrictive procedure. The stomach is staple to create a long vertical tube reduces the size of the stomach to 100 mL and therefore reducing the amount of calories one can consume. Unlike gastric bypass, this surgery does not alter the small bowel anatomy.

Gastric Sleeve

Gastric Pouch 30 mL

Excluded Stomach

Roux Limb 100 cm

Bilio-pancreatic Limb 100 cm

Common Channel

RYGB has two components. First, a small stomach pouch, approximately 30 mL in volume, is created by dividing the top of the stomach from the rest of the stomach. Next, the first portion of the small intestine is divided, and the bottom end of the divided small intestine is brought up and connected to the newly created small stomach pouch. The procedure is completed by connecting the top portion of the divided small intestine to the small intestine further down so that the stomach acids and digestive enzymes from the bypassed stomach and duodenum will eventually mix with the food.

Fig. 1. The 2 types of commonly performed bariatric procedures.

showed that the biliopancreatic diversion is more effective (99.0%) compared with RYGB (79.2%) in improving OSA.[70] This difference could be related to the greater degree of weight loss. A pooled analysis of metabolic surgical studies reported in 2012 showed that bariatric surgery offers a weighted decrease of BMI by 16 kg/m^2 (16.09; 95% CI, 13.27–18.92) and a weighted decrease of AHI by 34/h (34.22; 95% CI, 25.27–43.18).[10]

Preoperative screening of surgical patients for obstructive sleep apnea: judicious selection versus universal screening

Risk of OSA can be determined preoperatively with a focused history and careful clinical examination. Several of these have been validated for preoperative screening: the Berlin Questionnaire,[71] the American Society of Anesthesiologists checklist,[72] the STOP-Bang questionnaire,[73] and the Flemons index (Sleep Apnea Clinical Score).[74] If the risk of OSA is determined to be high, referral to a sleep specialist for preoperative polysomnography is recommended to further evaluate this risk.

Impact of obstructive sleep apnea on perioperative management

The role of OSA as a risk factor for anesthetic morbidity and mortality is considerable. The main perioperative risk factors associated with OSA include upper airway collapse, hypoxemia, and difficult airway control. Stierer and colleagues[75]

Table 2
Summary of changes in key hormones related to energy balance and weight for the established surgical procedures and for intentional dietary weight loss

	Adjustable Gastric Band	Sleeve Gastrectomy	Roux-en-Y Gastric Bypass	Biliopancreatic Diversion	Diet
Leptin	↓	↓	↓	↓	↓
Insulin	↓	↓	↓	↓	↓
Adiponectin	↑	↑	↑	↑	↑
Ghrelin	↑ ↔	↓	↓ ↔ ↑	↓	↑
GLP-1	↔	↑	↑	?	↔
peptide YY	?	↑	↑	↑	↔

↑ and ↓ indicate a substantial number of studies indicate an increase or decrease respectively; ↔ indicates a substantial number of studies find no change; and ? indicates that there are too few data to provide reliable trends.

Adapted from Dixon JB, Lambert EA, Lambert GW. Neuroendocrine adaptations to bariatric surgery. Mol Cell Endocrinol 2015;418 Pt 2:145; with permission; and *Data from* Sweeney TE, Morton JM. Metabolic surgery: action via hormonal milieu changes, changes in bile acids or gut microbiota? A summary of the literature. Best Pract Res Clin Gastroenterol 2014;28(4):727–40.

identified a difficult upper airway in 21.9% of OSA patients and in 2.6% of the controls, with intubation failure in 5% of the OSA patients. Some, but not all, data suggest that treatment of OSA with CPAP lead to a reduction of cardiovascular risk and mortality in these patients. Optimal preoperative benefit of CPAP may require greater than 1 month of treatment to allow the airway edema to subside.[76] In patients who have severe OSA or a significantly compromised airway, preoperative awake intubation and postoperative awake extubation is highly recommended to reduce airway collapse.[77] Reduction in anesthetic dose may also be helpful in patients who have OSA, and shorter-acting hypnotics may be preferred.[78,79] In those who have not used or been compliant with CPAP previously, or in undiagnosed cases, temporary introduction of CPAP until cessation of narcotic analgesic or sedative drugs is warranted.

When to do bariatric surgery for obstructive sleep apnea

According to the NIH guidelines, bariatric surgery is indicated for BMI of 35 kg/m^2 or more with OSA or other obesity-related complications.[80] Asians have higher risks of developing obesity-related complications at lower BMIs when compared with whites; hence, BMI cutoff for Asians is lowered to 32.5 kg/m^2.[81]

SUMMARY AND FINAL RECOMMENDATIONS

Like obesity, OSA is a chronic disease that is progressive if left untreated. Lifestyle modification with the aim of weight loss is fundamental to the treatment of both. Weight loss addresses the underlying pathophysiology of OSA and concurrently improves the concurrent obesity-associated diseases and reduces the CV risk factors, especially T2DM.

Weight loss of 7% to 11% as the initial and sole therapy can be considered for mild OSA. This can be achieved with lifestyle interventions alone or with adjunctive pharmacotherapy. For obese patients with moderate to severe OSA who cannot adhere to or tolerate CPAP treatment, more aggressive treatment combining lifestyle intervention, pharmacotherapy, and/or bariatric surgery should be considered. One treatment approach could be to place patients on short-term VCLD (8–12 weeks) followed by pharmacotherapy with liraglutide or combination phentermine–topiramate for further weight loss and maintenance.

Long-term studies 15 years postoperative have shown that bariatric surgery reduces mortality and CV events.[82] In morbidly obese individuals with more severe OSA, and multiple other obesity-related diseases in which greater weight loss with resolution or improvements in these conditions reduce total CV risk, bariatric surgery as a primary treatment should be strongly considered.

With the continued rise in obesity and its accompanied diseases, prevention is key. Public awareness, patient education, opportunistic screening with early detection, and initiation of therapy reduce the burden of obesity and OSA and its severity in the long-term. More interventions and health policies should be targeted in these aspects alongside clinical research for the optimal management of overweight and obesity in patients with OSA.[2]

REFERENCES

1. WHO. Obesity and overweight. 2018. Available at: http://www.who.int/news-room/fact-sheets/detail/obesity-and-overweight. Accessed July 25, 2018.
2. OECD. Obesity update. 2017. Available at: http://www.oecd.org/health/health-systems/Obesity-Update-2017.pdf. Accessed July 25, 2018.
3. Young T, Skatrud J, Peppard PE. Risk factors for obstructive sleep apnea in adults. JAMA 2004; 291(16):2013–6.
4. Lindberg E, Gislason T. Epidemiology of sleep-related obstructive breathing. Sleep Med Rev 2000;4(5):411–33.
5. Young T, Peppard PE, Taheri S. Excess weight and sleep-disordered breathing. J Appl Physiol (1985) 2005;99(4):1592–9.
6. Young T, Palta M, Dempsey J, et al. The occurrence of sleep-disordered breathing among middle-aged adults. N Engl J Med 1993;328(17):1230–5.
7. Peppard PE, Young T, Barnet JH, et al. Increased prevalence of sleep-disordered breathing in adults. Am J Epidemiol 2013;177(9):1006–14.
8. Collaboration NCDRF. Trends in adult body-mass index in 200 countries from 1975 to 2014: a pooled analysis of 1698 population-based measurement studies with 19.2 million participants. Lancet 2016; 387(10026):1377–96.
9. Pillar G, Shehadeh N. Abdominal fat and sleep apnea: the chicken or the egg? Diabetes Care 2008; 31(Suppl 2):S303–9.
10. Ashrafian H, le Roux CW, Rowland SP, et al. Metabolic surgery and obstructive sleep apnoea: the protective effects of bariatric procedures. Thorax 2012; 67(5):442–9.
11. Foster GD, Borradaile KE, Sanders MH, et al. A randomized study on the effect of weight loss on obstructive sleep apnea among obese patients with type 2 diabetes: the Sleep AHEAD study. Arch Intern Med 2009;169(17):1619–26.
12. Deflandre E, Gerdom A, Lamarque C, et al. Understanding pathophysiological concepts leading to obstructive apnea. Obes Surg 2018;28(8):2560–71.

13. Hardy OT, Czech MP, Corvera S. What causes the insulin resistance underlying obesity? Curr Opin Endocrinol Diabetes Obes 2012;19(2):81–7.

14. Sharma N, Lee J, Youssef I, et al. Obesity, cardiovascular disease and sleep disorders: insights into the rising epidemic. J Sleep Disord Ther 2017;6(1) [pii:260].

15. Ong CW, O'Driscoll DM, Truby H, et al. The reciprocal interaction between obesity and obstructive sleep apnoea. Sleep Med Rev 2013;17(2):123–31.

16. St-Onge MP. The role of sleep duration in the regulation of energy balance: effects on energy intakes and expenditure. J Clin Sleep Med 2013;9(1):73–80.

17. Spiegel K, Tasali E, Leproult R, et al. Effects of poor and short sleep on glucose metabolism and obesity risk. Nat Rev Endocrinol 2009;5(5):253–61.

18. Spiegel K, Tasali E, Penev P, et al. Brief communication: sleep curtailment in healthy young men is associated with decreased leptin levels, elevated ghrelin levels, and increased hunger and appetite. Ann Intern Med 2004;141(11):846–50.

19. Cefalu WT, Bray GA, Home PD, et al. Advances in the science, treatment, and prevention of the disease of obesity: reflections from a diabetes care editors' expert forum. Diabetes Care 2015;38(8):1567–82.

20. Garvey WT, Garber AJ, Mechanick JI, et al. American association of clinical endocrinologists and american college of endocrinology position statement on the 2014 advanced framework for a new diagnosis of obesity as a chronic disease. Endocr Pract 2014;20(9):977–89.

21. Magkos F, Fraterrigo G, Yoshino J, et al. Effects of moderate and subsequent progressive weight loss on metabolic function and adipose tissue biology in humans with obesity. Cell Metab 2016;23(4):591–601.

22. Jensen MD, Ryan DH, Apovian CM, et al. 2013 AHA/ACC/TOS guideline for the management of overweight and obesity in adults: a report of the American College of Cardiology/American Heart Association Task Force on Practice Guidelines and The Obesity Society. Circulation 2014;129(25 Suppl 2):S102–38.

23. Look ARG, Wing RR, Bolin P, et al. Cardiovascular effects of intensive lifestyle intervention in type 2 diabetes. N Engl J Med 2013;369(2):145–54.

24. Johansson K, Neovius M, Lagerros YT, et al. Effect of a very low energy diet on moderate and severe obstructive sleep apnoea in obese men: a randomised controlled trial. BMJ 2009;339:b4609.

25. Kuna ST, Reboussin DM, Borradaile KE, et al. Long-term effect of weight loss on obstructive sleep apnea severity in obese patients with type 2 diabetes. Sleep 2013;36(5):641–649A.

26. Peromaa-Haavisto P, Tuomilehto H, Kossi J, et al. Obstructive sleep apnea: the effect of bariatric surgery after 12 months. A prospective multicenter trial. Sleep Med 2017;35:85–90.

27. Araghi MH, Chen YF, Jagielski A, et al. Effectiveness of lifestyle interventions on obstructive sleep apnea (OSA): systematic review and meta-analysis. Sleep 2013;36(10):1553–62, 1562A–1562E.

28. Tuomilehto HP, Seppa JM, Partinen MM, et al. Lifestyle intervention with weight reduction: first-line treatment in mild obstructive sleep apnea. Am J Respir Crit Care Med 2009;179(4):320–7.

29. Johnston BC, Kanters S, Bandayrel K, et al. Comparison of weight loss among named diet programs in overweight and obese adults: a meta-analysis. JAMA 2014;312(9):923–33.

30. Franz MJ, VanWormer JJ, Crain AL, et al. Weight-loss outcomes: a systematic review and meta-analysis of weight-loss clinical trials with a minimum 1-year follow-up. J Am Diet Assoc 2007;107(10):1755–67.

31. Tsai AG, Wadden TA. The evolution of very-low-calorie diets: an update and meta-analysis. Obesity (Silver Spring) 2006;14(8):1283–93.

32. Purcell K, Sumithran P, Prendergast LA, et al. The effect of rate of weight loss on long-term weight management: a randomised controlled trial. Lancet Diabetes Endocrinol 2014;2(12):954–62.

33. Kansanen M, Vanninen E, Tuunainen A, et al. The effect of a very low-calorie diet-induced weight loss on the severity of obstructive sleep apnoea and autonomic nervous function in obese patients with obstructive sleep apnoea syndrome. Clin Physiol 1998;18(4):377–85.

34. Johansson K, Hemmingsson E, Harlid R, et al. Longer term effects of very low energy diet on obstructive sleep apnoea in cohort derived from randomised controlled trial: prospective observational follow-up study. BMJ 2011;342:d3017.

35. Willett WC, Sacks F, Trichopoulou A, et al. Mediterranean diet pyramid: a cultural model for healthy eating. Am J Clin Nutr 1995;61(6 Suppl):1402S–6S.

36. Estruch R, Ros E, Salas-Salvado J, et al. Primary prevention of cardiovascular disease with a Mediterranean diet. N Engl J Med 2013;368(14):1279–90.

37. Salas-Salvado J, Bullo M, Babio N, et al. Reduction in the incidence of type 2 diabetes with the Mediterranean diet: results of the PREDIMED-Reus nutrition intervention randomized trial. Diabetes Care 2011;34(1):14–9.

38. Kastorini CM, Milionis HJ, Esposito K, et al. The effect of Mediterranean diet on metabolic syndrome and its components: a meta-analysis of 50 studies and 534,906 individuals. J Am Coll Cardiol 2011;57(11):1299–313.

39. Sofi F, Casini A. Mediterranean diet and non-alcoholic fatty liver disease: new therapeutic option around the corner? World J Gastroenterol 2014; 20(23):7339–46.

40. Papandreou C, Schiza SE, Bouloukaki I, et al. Effect of Mediterranean diet versus prudent diet combined with physical activity on OSAS: a randomised trial. Eur Respir J 2012;39(6):1398–404.

41. Dobrosielski DA, Papandreou C, Patil SP, et al. Diet and exercise in the management of obstructive sleep apnoea and cardiovascular disease risk. Eur Respir Rev 2017;26(144) [pii: 160110].

42. Haskell WL, Lee IM, Pate RR, et al. Physical activity and public health: updated recommendation for adults from the American College of Sports Medicine and the American Heart Association. Circulation 2007;116(9):1081–93.

43. Warburton DE, Nicol CW, Bredin SS. Health benefits of physical activity: the evidence. CMAJ 2006; 174(6):801–9.

44. Santos RV, Tufik S, De Mello MT. Exercise, sleep and cytokines: is there a relation? Sleep Med Rev 2007; 11(3):231–9.

45. Kline CE, Crowley EP, Ewing GB, et al. The effect of exercise training on obstructive sleep apnea and sleep quality: a randomized controlled trial. Sleep 2011;34(12):1631–40.

46. Netzer N, Lormes W, Giebelhaus V, et al. Physical training of patients with sleep apnea. Pneumologie 1997;51(Suppl 3):779–82 [in German].

47. Giebelhaus V, Strohl KP, Lormes W, et al. Physical exercise as an adjunct therapy in sleep apnea-an open trial. Sleep Breath 2000;4(4):173–6.

48. Redolfi S, Bettinzoli M, Venturoli N, et al. Attenuation of obstructive sleep apnea and overnight rostral fluid shift by physical activity. Am J Respir Crit Care Med 2015;191(7):856–8.

49. Borel AL, Leblanc X, Almeras N, et al. Sleep apnoea attenuates the effects of a lifestyle intervention programme in men with visceral obesity. Thorax 2012; 67(8):735–41.

50. Stamatakis KA, Punjabi NM. Effects of sleep fragmentation on glucose metabolism in normal subjects. Chest 2010;137(1):95–101.

51. Quan SF, Budhiraja R, Clarke DP, et al. Impact of treatment with continuous positive airway pressure (CPAP) on weight in obstructive sleep apnea. J Clin Sleep Med 2013;9(10):989–93.

52. Kajaste S, Brander PE, Telakivi T, et al. A cognitive-behavioral weight reduction program in the treatment of obstructive sleep apnea syndrome with or without initial nasal CPAP: a randomized study. Sleep Med 2004;5(2):125–31.

53. Chirinos JA, Gurubhagavatula I, Teff K, et al. CPAP, weight loss, or both for obstructive sleep apnea. N Engl J Med 2014;370(24):2265–75.

54. Sumithran P, Prendergast LA, Delbridge E, et al. Long-term persistence of hormonal adaptations to weight loss. N Engl J Med 2011;365(17):1597–604.

55. Rosenbaum M, Hirsch J, Gallagher DA, et al. Long-term persistence of adaptive thermogenesis in subjects who have maintained a reduced body weight. Am J Clin Nutr 2008;88(4):906–12.

56. Apovian CM, Garvey WT, Ryan DH. Challenging obesity: patient, provider, and expert perspectives on the roles of available and emerging nonsurgical therapies. Obesity (Silver Spring) 2015;23(Suppl 2):S1–26.

57. Apovian CM, Aronne LJ, Bessesen DH, et al. Pharmacological management of obesity: an endocrine Society clinical practice guideline. J Clin Endocrinol Metab 2015;100(2):342–62.

58. Garcia Hernandez E, Gonzalez Rodriguez JL, Vega Cruz MS. Cesarean delivery and exeresis of a pheochromocytoma performed under epidural and general anesthesia. Rev Esp Anestesiol Reanim 2004; 51(4):217–20 [in Spanish].

59. Winslow DH, Bowden CH, DiDonato KP, et al. A randomized, double-blind, placebo-controlled study of an oral, extended-release formulation of phentermine/topiramate for the treatment of obstructive sleep apnea in obese adults. Sleep 2012; 35(11):1529–39.

60. Blackman A, Foster GD, Zammit G, et al. Effect of liraglutide 3.0 mg in individuals with obesity and moderate or severe obstructive sleep apnea: the SCALE Sleep Apnea randomized clinical trial. Int J Obes 2016;40(8):1310–9.

61. Davies MJ, Bergenstal R, Bode B, et al. Efficacy of liraglutide for weight loss among patients with type 2 diabetes: the SCALE diabetes randomized clinical trial. JAMA 2015;314(7):687–99.

62. Marso SP, Daniels GH, Brown-Frandsen K, et al. Liraglutide and cardiovascular outcomes in type 2 diabetes. N Engl J Med 2016;375(4):311–22.

63. Yanovski SZ, Yanovski JA. Long-term drug treatment for obesity: a systematic and clinical review. JAMA 2014;311(1):74–86.

64. Lee SY, Lim CH, Pasupathy S, et al. Laparoscopic sleeve gastrectomy: a novel procedure for weight loss. Singapore Med J 2011;52(11):794–800.

65. Lim CH, Jahansouz C, Abraham AA, et al. The future of the Roux-en-Y gastric bypass. Expert Rev Gastroenterol Hepatol 2016;10(7):777–84.

66. Buchwald H, Estok R, Fahrbach K, et al. Weight and type 2 diabetes after bariatric surgery: systematic review and meta-analysis. Am J Med 2009;122(3): 248–56.e5.

67. Sjostrom L, Narbro K, Sjostrom CD, et al. Effects of bariatric surgery on mortality in Swedish obese subjects. N Engl J Med 2007;357(8):741–52.

68. Toh BC, Chan WH, Eng AKH, et al. Five-year long-term clinical outcome after bariatric metabolic

surgery: a multi-ethnic Asian population in Singapore. Diabetes Obes Metab 2018;20(7): 1762–5.

69. Fredheim JM, Rollheim J, Sandbu R, et al. Obstructive sleep apnea after weight loss: a clinical trial comparing gastric bypass and intensive lifestyle intervention. J Clin Sleep Med 2013;9(5):427–32.

70. Sarkhosh K, Switzer NJ, El-Hadi M, et al. The impact of bariatric surgery on obstructive sleep apnea: a systematic review. Obes Surg 2013;23(3):414–23.

71. Chung F, Yegneswaran B, Liao P, et al. Validation of the Berlin questionnaire and American Society of Anesthesiologists checklist as screening tools for obstructive sleep apnea in surgical patients. Anesthesiology 2008;108(5):822–30.

72. Gross JB, Bachenberg KL, Benumof JL, et al. Practice guidelines for the perioperative management of patients with obstructive sleep apnea: a report by the American Society of Anesthesiologists Task Force on Perioperative Management of patients with obstructive sleep apnea. Anesthesiology 2006;104(5):1081–93 [quiz: 1117–8].

73. Chung F, Yegneswaran B, Liao P, et al. STOP questionnaire: a tool to screen patients for obstructive sleep apnea. Anesthesiology 2008; 108(5):812–21.

74. Flemons WW, Whitelaw WA, Brant R, et al. Likelihood ratios for a sleep apnea clinical prediction rule. Am J Respir Crit Care Med 1994;150(5 Pt 1):1279–85.

75. Stierer TL, Wright C, George A, et al. Risk assessment of obstructive sleep apnea in a population of patients undergoing ambulatory surgery. J Clin Sleep Med 2010;6(5):467–72.

76. Seet E, Chung F. Management of sleep apnea in adults - functional algorithms for the perioperative period: continuing professional development. Can J Anaesth 2010;57(9):849–64.

77. Lan CK, Rose MW. Perioperative management of obstructive sleep apnea. Sleep Med Clin 2006;1: 541–8.

78. Pawlik MT, Hansen E, Waldhauser D, et al. Clonidine premedication in patients with sleep apnea syndrome: a randomized, double-blind, placebo-controlled study. Anesth Analg 2005;101(5): 1374–80.

79. Liu SS, Chisholm MF, Ngeow J, et al. Postoperative hypoxemia in orthopedic patients with obstructive sleep apnea. HSS J 2011;7(1):2–8.

80. NIH conference. Gastrointestinal surgery for severe obesity. Consensus development conference panel. Ann Intern Med 1991;115(12):956–61.

81. WHO Expert Consultation. Appropriate body-mass index for Asian populations and its implications for policy and intervention strategies. Lancet 2004; 363(9403):157–63.

82. Sjostrom L, Peltonen M, Jacobson P, et al. Bariatric surgery and long-term cardiovascular events. JAMA 2012;307(1):56–65.

Moving?

Make sure your subscription moves with you!

To notify us of your new address, find your **Clinics Account Number** (located on your mailing label above your name), and contact customer service at:

Email: journalscustomerservice-usa@elsevier.com

800-654-2452 (subscribers in the U.S. & Canada)
314-447-8871 (subscribers outside of the U.S. & Canada)

Fax number: 314-447-8029

Elsevier Health Sciences Division
Subscription Customer Service
3251 Riverport Lane
Maryland Heights, MO 63043

*To ensure uninterrupted delivery of your subscription, please notify us at least 4 weeks in advance of move.